D1570292

When I began reading *Designed to Heal*, I felt the same flush of excitement that I had when I first encountered Dr. Paul Brand, my collaborator on three books. These two authors, a researcher and a physician, have woven together a rare combination of vivid science, compassionate storytelling, and lasting spiritual lessons. A delight to read.

PHILIP YANCEY, bestselling author

To work in prison ministry is to see, day in and day out, the damage that unhealed wounds can create in a life and a community. This book paints a vivid picture of the hope we share—that God's love can bring healing to even the most profound of wounds, and the mechanisms through which that healing may come to pass.

JED BREWER, director of productions at Mission:USA

I have tried to come up with just the right word to describe this book, and the best I can do is "marvelous." Medical doctor Jennie McLaurin, with the help of her friend, molecular geneticist Cymbeline Culiat, has written a marvelous book. They open up for us the wonders of the human body, in particular the marvel of the body's inherent capacity for healing. I was stunned by what they show us: the ability of the body to repair, restore, and even regenerate. Drs. McLaurin and Culiat take us through the remarkable stages by which such wound healing takes place and apply them to the healing of corporate bodies, especially the church, the body of Christ. Through their stories of healing, clear and easily grasped biological explanations, and solid theological insights, I find myself lifted into hope that *all* wounds can be healed, and one day will be. Marvelous in every sense of the word!

DARRELL JOHNSON, retired pastor and professor, teaching fellow at Regent College, and theological mentor

This is a book of hope—hope in the grace that courses through our healing physical bodies and for the communal bodies that we live among. The wonders of science, illuminated by a physician and a molecular geneticist, shed light on possibilities for families, neighborhoods, churches, and the body politic. Drs. McLaurin and Culiat are close friends who share deep commitments to science, motherhood, and living out their Christian faith in our complicated world. Acknowledging the reality of woundedness, physical and social, they offer ways of seeing and living that will bless the world.

> SUSAN S. PHILLIPS, PHD, executive director of New College Berkeley, sociologist, and author of *The Crisis of Care* (with Patricia Benner) and *The Cultivated Life*

This unique and very interesting book examines the processes by which our bodies heal, and applies that learning to the healing of relationships. The authors share current brain science research relating to the damaging effects of trauma and the protective effects of positive emotions and experiences. Overall a very valuable and useful new perspective.

> BRIAN ALLAIN, founder of Writing for Your Life and How to Heal Our Divides

The prevalence and intensity of current conflicts in personal and communal lives have reached critical levels globally. This book presents a refreshing and intriguing new perspective on how the injuries in our lives can heal by applying the principles of how the physical body naturally heals wounds. Combining scientific and medical knowledge with engaging stories from the clinic, the laboratory, and their personal lives, the authors have crafted a unique work that has great potential to bring healing to the injured spaces of any reader's life.

> LISA GOKONGWEI-CHENG, president of Summit Media, Manila, Philippines

On this fascinating journey, two medical friends invite readers into the human body's capacity to heal its physical wounds and provide a spiritual blueprint for healing our broken communities. Kind, savvy, and encouraging, pediatrician Jennie McLaurin and scientist Cymbeline Tancongco Culiat apply the balm of insight, story, and encouragement to inspire fresh ways of exploring how God's people and our connections can be healed and also transformed. It's a restorative adventure worth taking.

PATRICIA RAYBON, author of *My First White Friend: Confessions on Race, Love, and Forgiveness* and *I Told the Mountain to Move: Learning to Pray So Things Change*

In this engaging book, a physician and a scientist share their stories of injury and healing. As they describe the amazing biological processes at work in our physical bodies, we gain new insights into ways to promote healing in our relationships, churches, and communities. A timely book, excellent for preachers, small groups, and our wounded world.

DEBORAH HAARSMA, president of BioLogos

We are indeed spiritual beings in physical bodies that God created with amazing healing capabilities. God in his glory and majesty created our bodies magnificently, and *Designed to Heal* gives us a glimpse of what we can learn from the wondrous design of physical healing and what it teaches us about how to experience relational and emotional healing as well. It marries scientific and spiritual understanding to give a visual presentation of the work needed for us to be completely restored and transformed—not only from our physical wounds but also from our emotional, relational, and spiritual wounds as individuals and as one body of Christ. I recommend that you read this book and hope that it blesses you!

DR. PETER TAN-CHI, senior pastor, Christ's Commission Fellowship

McLaurin and Culiat thoughtfully compare the biological processes of wound healing to the steps needed to heal the human soul, what the Greeks called our psyche. Although biological healing appears to be spontaneous and almost miraculous (even to the medical community), healing our hearts requires more intervention. Whether it is our individual psyche or the corporate psyche of our families and communities, the authors provide practical examples (many from their own lives) that can encourage and enable us to seek the healing that leads to wholeness. I wholeheartedly recommend this book as one I will share with friends and family.

ROGER E. STOLLER, PHD, distinguished materials scientist, Oak Ridge National Laboratory (retired)

DESIGNED *to* HEAL

DESIGNED

to

HEAL

WHAT THE BODY SHOWS US

ABOUT HEALING WOUNDS,

REPAIRING RELATIONSHIPS,

AND RESTORING COMMUNITY

☞

Jennie A. McLaurin

Cymbeline Tancongco Culiat

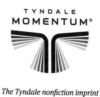

TYNDALE
MOMENTUM®

The Tyndale nonfiction imprint

Visit Tyndale online at tyndale.com.

Visit Tyndale Momentum online at tyndalemomentum.com.

TYNDALE, Tyndale's quill logo, *Tyndale Momentum*, and the Tyndale Momentum logo are registered trademarks of Tyndale House Ministries. Tyndale Momentum is the nonfiction imprint of Tyndale House Publishers, Carol Stream, Illinois.

Designed by Koko Toyama

Published in association with the literary agency of WordServe Literary Group, www.wordserveliterary.com.

For information about special discounts for bulk purchases, please contact Tyndale House Publishers at csresponse@tyndale.com, or call 1-855-277-9400.

Library of Congress Cataloging-in-Publication Data

Names: McLaurin, Jennie A., author. | Culiat, Cymbeline Tancongco, author.
Title: Designed to heal : what the body shows us about healing wounds, repairing relationships, and restoring community / Jennie A. McLaurin and Cymbeline Tancongco Culiat.
Description: Carol Stream, Illinois : Tyndale House Publishers, [2021] | Includes bibliographical references.
Identifiers: LCCN 2021004324 (print) | LCCN 2021004325 (ebook) | ISBN 9781496447791 (hardcover) | ISBN 9781496447814 (kindle edition) | ISBN 9781496447821 (epub) | ISBN 9781496447838 (epub)
Subjects: LCSH: Emotions--Psychological aspects. | Mind and body. | Interpersonal relations.
Classification: LCC BF511 .M33 2021 (print) | LCC BF511 (ebook) | DDC 152.4—dc23
LC record available at https://lccn.loc.gov/2021004324
LC ebook record available at https://lccn.loc.gov/2021004325

Printed in the United States of America

27	26	25	24	23	22	21
7	6	5	4	3	2	1

To the faithful restorers and
sustainers of our healing matrix:
Andrew, Luci, and Larry
Julio and Caleb

CONTENTS

FOREWORD

FIFTEEN YEARS AGO Dr. Jennie McLaurin blew into my life like a fresh wind. I first met her when she took a journal-writing course that I was teaching at Regent College in Vancouver, British Columbia. From that early introduction I remember well her energy and her vivid personality.

I come from a family of physicians—two grandfathers, father, brother, son—and while I'm not a doctor myself, I feel a kindred spirit with healers and professionals like Jennie McLaurin and her colleague and friend Cymbeline (Bem) Culiat, who can investigate the causes and cures of physical wounds and diseases. As a mother of five, I've also learned a lot over the years, sometimes by painful experience, about illness and accidents, pain and healing.

My father was a surgeon, a medical missionary in the Solomon Islands. After his retirement, the family moved to England, where my brother and I were born. We were his only children. Under his influence we lived a life full of adventures and challenges, both physical and spiritual, eventually relocating to Australia. To my mother's panicked horror, he would challenge us to test our limits, climbing cliffs, hiking and bushwhacking through forests, swimming in the breakers along rocky beaches. On one such outing I cut my ankle on a sharp oyster shell. I remember how freely it bled and eventually healed under the bandages, though it left a four-inch scar. This was, of course, back in the 1940s, before the widespread use of antibiotics.

My father was a born optimist, and when we would come to him sobbing after a fall or a cut, his invariable treatment advice was, "Nothing to worry about. Dab it with peroxide. Then put some baby powder on it to make a scab. It'll heal under the scab, but don't pick at it or pull it off, or it might get infected."

So we would dab our scrapes with hydrogen peroxide and watch the little wound fizz, thinking, *Aha! It's working!*

Now, many years later, new understandings of the healing process are being applied, and that's when this remarkable book by Jennie and Bem has arrived, with groundbreaking revelations. I'd heard from these two experts about their fresh understandings of the stages of wound healing, and I was privileged to read an early version of this manuscript. As I read, I grew more and more excited about the fascinating details of the process and how relational as well as physical healing can happen. I encouraged these friends to disclose this information to a wider public, to show us how the metaphor of the physical healing mechanism can be applied in damaged human relationships to ease tension, heal hurts, and mend the divisions that are prevalent in human nature and in communities of faith.

I remember how, several years ago, during a drive to a weekend getaway with Jennie and Bem, we three engaged in a long and fruitful conversation about how this process of healing and recovery might be applied. The context was not just a discussion about a therapy for physical wounds but a more comprehensive vision of how this intricate process of healing and recovery might be applied to fractures within personal and community relationships that have become toxic because of conflicts, either perceived or imagined.

As a poet and writer, I value all fresh and creative insight into the human condition. During that weekend conversation I felt so energized that I insisted that these insights be written about and published. I told them I'd do anything to encourage that process, to make it a book. They have taken me up on that, and because their thinking and insights are so original, so powerful, I am convinced that this unique book will have a profound impact.

I've come to depend on my friendship with Jennie, who is a wise, supportive friend and clinician. And I'm deeply grateful and excited, now, to be recommending Jennie and Bem's book to the wider world where the vital healing of bodies and souls is so desperately needed.

Go with God, Jennie and Bem. We'll hear you and follow along!

Luci Shaw
Poet and Writer-in-Residence at Regent College,
Vancouver, British Columbia

BODIES

by Jennie A. McLaurin

*The human body has been called the microcosm of
the universe, a little world of wonders and a monument
of divine wisdom and power, sufficient to convince the most
incredulous mind of the existence of the Great Designer.*

A. B. SIMPSON

DESPITE SAYING FOR YEARS that they wouldn't put a bumper
sticker on a Bentley, my sons recently got tattoos together.
Knowing I would worry about the hygiene of the techniques
used, the permanency of the choice, and the meaning of the
design, they chose to surprise me. The family crest spreads
across a forearm of the older and a thigh of the younger. After
the boys endured a few days of swelling, redness, and mild
pain, the images became background art instead of acute
injuries. They are delighted with their choices, and I am still
thrilled to be their mom.

Actually, I frequently find tattoos during the physical
exams I do every Tuesday in an adolescent clinic. Sometimes
the images are just flowers or abstract designs. Other times

they are pop culture icons or the names of loved ones. Often when a patient shares their meaning, I get a lump in my throat.

Elijah's exam is one I particularly recall.[1] He greeted me with a broad smile and an open expression. I could see a block letter tattoo on his neck as I shook his hand but couldn't decipher the words. Eagerly, he shared how he was going to study nursing after completing his high school requirements. This program was a new start, he said, a chance to better his opportunities.

As I spoke with Elijah about any past hospitalizations, he told me of two. One was for facial reconstruction. I glanced more closely at his face, amazed that I could see no trace of a scar. He grinned, saying he had an awesome surgeon. Why did he need reconstruction? I wondered. Elijah replied with two words—*brass knuckles*. Then he balled up his fist and put it over his left eye.

Talking on, Elijah said he was so fortunate to have full sight and a symmetrical face after his left orbital bones were fractured in a gang-related fight. He moved away from that crowd after his surgeries, but his hospitalizations weren't over. When he started seeing and hearing things that others didn't and became frightened of going anywhere in public, he was diagnosed with schizophrenia. Another month of his life was spent in a medical ward, and now he was left with a problem that couldn't be fixed in an operating room. His medicines helped him feel functional again, but he said he still saw and heard things. He had learned, so far anyway, to cope with them as background noise.

Elijah's physical body seemed to be in great shape. He was slender with a muscular frame; I checked all the boxes "Normal" on the physical form. At the conclusion of the visit, I asked Elijah what the tattoo on his neck said.

"Resilient," he replied.

As a physician, I'm an expert on the bodies I encounter in the exam room. But even there, I'm often struck by how ill-equipped I am to remedy life's complex wounds, like the distressing emotional ones suffered by Elijah. Just like the human body that I know so well from medical training, the corporate bodies I inhabit—whether my church, my family, or my workplace—are sometimes healthy and sometimes injured. We all want our collective bodies to stay well, but many times those wounds also appear too complicated to heal.

Family strains, workplace stress, church policy disagreements, and world politics have all taken a toll on my well-being. And the problem isn't just "them"—it is me as well. How do I respond as my authentic self in times of stress, crisis, and deep hurt? When should I let go of a conflict and when should I hang on, pushing for a better resolution? Am I hurting or helping? These problems are harder for me to solve than most of my pediatric cases.

Our physical bodies are designed to heal, even when faced with extraordinary circumstances. Our healing tendencies are integrated into every system of the body, responsive down to the most basic microcellular level. As humans, we will all experience hurt; indeed, woundedness is part of what it means to be alive. But due to the amazing design of our bodies, our injuries don't have to have the last word. Repair, restoration, and even regeneration are built into our very cells. In fact, the actual healing process is complex, involving distinct stages and many cell types that contribute to the overall work in an orderly, patient progression.

What if our corporate bodies were oriented to healing the way our physical bodies are? People of Abrahamic faiths see our bodies as made in the image of God. That image can extend down to the holistic engagement of our microcellular properties toward restoration and renewal. Likewise, Christians call ourselves the body of Christ. That term is a collective one—literally, a corporate one—encompassing all of us in a mysterious unbreakable bond of unity in diversity. And so we may draw on the analogy between the human body's natural wound-healing system and the ways we can mirror those processes as we strive to heal communal wounds, whether in the church, the family, the workplace, or the wider community.

This fresh portrayal of how we heal is written from the context of what C. S. Lewis termed *mere Christianity*. It is grounded in traditional understandings of faith with a generosity toward interpretations of doctrine and expression. As our physical healing depends upon a diverse array of actors, so this representation acknowledges the helpful roles of a variety of healers, including some outside the confines of the church or faith communities.

Let's look a little closer at wound healing, whether of a tattoo or a major trauma. We all know at least a bit of the science of wound healing just by our life experiences. Our knees get scraped and blood oozes out. Soon it is sticky and a bit darker red. We might put on a Band-Aid. Later, we look to see if a scab has formed, but so far there is some pink tissue at the edges and yellow gummy stuff in the middle. We put on a new bandage and wait a few days. By then there is a hard scab. We try to leave it alone until it unroofs to reveal bright pink, tender new skin. Later, we may have a faint scar if the wound was deep or if we kept annoying the scab. Those observations are the macro-level stories of wound healing. In the chapters ahead we will travel inside the body and see what happens on the micro level.

While it may seem wonderful enough that our body stops bleeding and makes a scab, seeing the world of wound healing at the micro level is more captivating than any Pixar film could portray. Through four separate stages, the wounds of our physical bodies are replaced by new structures—blood vessels, skin, and nerves—a truly transformational process. It is one of the most studied and highly orchestrated biological processes known in science. Over and over again, scientists refer to it as a beautifully choreographed system. Its precision coupled with complexity fascinates both students and experts.

Attending to healing, in all aspects of our gathered lives, is not just for those with special gifts, but is a call that encompasses everyone. Through exploring the science of wound healing, we see in more depth what it means to be a body, how fully formed we are toward collaboration and wholeness, and how much we depend on processes designed to protect our health. This reflection gives us new ways of seeing how emotional and spiritual wounds with our neighbors can be more fully healed. This book is meant to bring light and a way forward to anyone stuck in the pain of their life journey. It is also a companion for all who walk alongside those who suffer.

A SHARED MISSION

I've never met anyone with a career quite like mine. I am a pediatrician with master's degrees in public health and in theology and culture. As such, I juggle several sorts of jobs at any one time. Clinical practice, teaching, writing, research, and consulting fill my weeks. For more than thirty years, I've worked with marginalized communities in public health settings, serving immigrants, migrant farmworker families, native Hawaiians, and homeless youth in America and abroad. Currently, I split my clinical work between a special-needs center for infants and toddlers and an adolescent center for vulnerable youth. The gift of this unusual career has been to witness many cultures, family situations, and health conditions in deeply personal settings. Faith and medicine are inseparable for me, as both animate who I am as I engage in this world.

An extraordinary gift of my work has been the colleagues I've come to treasure. Cymbeline (Bem) Culiat, a renowned researcher in molecular genetics, is one such friend. We met at a bioethics conference I was leading. Our conversation went quickly from simple greetings to delighted discussion that spilled over into the rest of the weekend. Bem expressed ideas about ethics, science, and wonder that encouraged and captivated me. Our shared faith added depth and breadth to the ideas we pondered. When I received an international grant aimed at helping church leaders engage with science as a positive aspect of pastoral ministry, Bem became a partner and mentor to the pastors. As the years have passed, we have become connected not just through our professional interests, but through shared stories of family, joy, grief, and hope. Bem and I see through a lens shaped by science and medicine. While I am a physician, Bem is a molecular geneticist who specializes in tissue repair and regeneration research. Her knowledge enables people to recover more fully from their diseases and transforms the methods doctors use in caring for patients. Together, Bem and I attend to biochemical processes and seek to promote wholeness and healing from the laboratory to the bedside.

We understand our careers as callings, an ongoing witness to the revelation of God's dwelling among us. This calling shapes our identity as women of faith and our understanding of how God manifests himself in this world.

One way in which God reveals his splendor is through the way our body heals its wounds—a process so ordinary and universal that we almost never notice it happening and yet so orderly and intricate that parts of it still defy understanding. Most physicians are not as familiar with wound healing as research scientists like Bem. My own wound science education was long ago, and what I remember most clearly is the professor of surgery silently writing across the chalkboard: *On the Fifth Day God Made Pus!* He wanted us to remember that infections usually popped up about five days after surgery, so if a patient had a fever then, we were to examine the wound. All clinicians know that each phase of wound healing has a precise order and process that must be followed, or healing will be delayed and complicated by difficult problems.

Bem introduced me to the wonder and complexity of healing at the microcellular level during a devotional she led in a group retreat. It wasn't a typical talk; Bem spoke with affection about mice, DNA, and wounded tissues. She painted a picture of a microscopic drama, filled with urgency, risk, rescue, and possibility. Death and life were tied up together—both had roles to play, and wholeness required both individual and communal participation. The healing process had to faithfully follow its God-given design, or all sorts of maladies would ensue. The other attendees and I were rapt, seeing new patterns we might embrace to transform our conflicts with others into reconciled relationships.

The intricate phases of wound healing that Bem described, I realized, take on flesh in my patients. Her world is made visible in mine. That devotional became a story to ponder. What does it mean to be made in the image of God? Do even our body's microprocesses reflect that image? And how does that affect the way we interact with one another?

IMAGINING A RESTORED WORLD

Imagination—a word derived from *image*. This is a book of Christian imagination. It is a journey through the body's extraordinary capacity for wound healing, which occurs in the four precisely ordered stages we'll introduce in chapter 1. We bring this process to life through the stories of patients. The book is a collection of medical parables, given in companionship with reflections on how we might better heal the wounds of our hurting world. Like all good parables, these stories are meant to provoke personal understandings rather than uniform interpretations.

As Bem and I considered how we might communicate what our physical bodies have to teach us about healing wounds within community, we were reminded of the parables told by Jesus. He used imagery from his everyday life as he shared his messages of hope and healing. Wheat, chaff, lost coins, lost sheep, wells, and wedding feasts were all subjects of his stories. They were familiar, but new twists gave meaning to issues like the kingdom of God and the patience of grace. The apostle Paul also used metaphors, comparing the life of faith to a race and the church to the human body. Despite the repeated use of body imagery and creation stories in the Bible, I've rarely heard a science-filled message in a local church. Perhaps many Christians haven't thought of scientific and spiritual understandings as being interrelated. Frequently, people think of science as difficult, or as a topic for a select few. Yet as Bem and I have considered how healing occurs in our human bodies and our broader relationships, we have noticed several parallels.

First, healing is a dynamic process that requires many changes. When the human body is wounded, everything from the blood vessels to the skin must go through a transformation. Likewise, healing within community requires an openness to change, to challenge, to revision, and to expansion. Ultimately, it may even change our ideas about suffering and hope as we work through the slow and painful process of acknowledging an injury and accepting change before being transformed into a newly functional body.

Second, physical healing happens only within cellular community, and emotional or spiritual healing also happens best in community. Finally, healing requires great perseverance. It always takes longer than we wish. We have to journey through several stages . . . and each one serves a purpose to ensure that real healing and restoration are achieved. Getting stuck in one phase or skipping a step in the process only results in more disability.

To illuminate the similarities between healing within the human body and within corporate bodies, each chapter starts with a tale from science and medicine—the anecdotes are true though real names are not used, and some are an amalgamation of patient stories. I am the book's primary writer, so narratives about patients and personal references are mine unless specifically noted. As coauthor, Bem supplied the scientific understandings of wound healing as well as many of the illustrations used in application. As we wrote, we recognized that it was not only our patients who provided us with windows into healing pathways, but our own experiences as well. During our partnership on this book, Bem and I both navigated times of personal need, loved ones' critical illnesses, strained relationships with family members, and the seemingly constant presence of conflict in the world around us. We have had an opportunity to try on these images—to practice what we preach—and in turn, to experience healing in hopeful new ways.

Most chapters explain the processes that are important to one or two particular phases of healing, as well as what can go awry during each critical step. As we explore each stage of wound healing, we will consider how we might apply a similar understanding to promote healing in our places of shared woundedness. Those who want to engage further with each chapter and see how the stages of wound healing might play out during one family's conflict will want to refer to the discussion guide at the back of the book. The story and discussion questions are designed to help readers consider how they might contribute to healing within their families, workplaces, churches, or other communities.

Bem and I are not counselors or therapists, and we do not want to make science a therapy tool. But science is a gift of common grace, as theologian and public figure Abraham Kuyper put it, and it can reveal truths that give life, both to our bodies and to the communities in which we live. Science, properly understood, should strengthen faith, not diminish it.

For people of Abrahamic faiths, there is a coherence to everything that is. A divine Creator made the world and all the universes that there may be. Kuyper encouraged people to look for connections in the universe that allowed them to see images of the Creator. He was concerned that we'd lost our understanding of creation's harmony—the integration of the whole, or the "divine thinking . . . embedded in all created things."[2]

Mysteriously, we echo that concept as we consider the Trinity. The Christian God is one yet three, separate yet in a reciprocal dance that cannot be divided or destroyed. Likewise, as human beings we are never really complete as individuals. From infancy to death, we rely on the attention of others for our physical, emotional, and spiritual well-being. We are shaped by social forces that are the undercurrent of our communities, often not even recognizing their role in our formation. Parents sacrifice self for their children, faith communities experience growth in gathered worship, and rituals mark our care of the dying. Whether in our corporate bodies or our individual ones, signals we don't fully comprehend call us to one another, to link us together through a process that shapes us to fit the form and function of shalom.

Although you won't become an expert in all things medical after reading this book, you will marvel at the interconnectedness and precision of each phase of healing—whether in your own body or the collective body of your family, faith community, school, neighborhood, or workplace. But unlike in your school science lab, you will need no protective equipment to enter this scientific space; all you need is to stay open to wonder, delight, and curiosity.

CHAPTER I

WOUNDED

The Four Phases of Healing

In a world so torn apart by rivalry, anger, and hatred,
we have the privileged vocation to be living signs of a love
that can bridge all divisions and heal all wounds.

HENRI NOUWEN

YEARS AGO MY FAMILY went for a sunny day trip to Mt. Baker, the volcanic peak just sixty miles from our home in north-western Washington State. At almost 11,000 feet high, its glaciers glisten year-round. On that bright July day, a basin near the winter ski area was filled with snow. We couldn't wait to share summer sledding with my husband's family, who were visiting from North Carolina. Everyone took turns tumbling down the steep hill on a floppy plastic sled. Andrew, my husband, hopped on for the last ride of the day. We laughingly warned him to avoid the one stick popping up in the otherwise smooth, snowy meadow below.

Somehow, Andrew careened straight into that stick. After

hitting it, he flew up in the air with the sled and came down sprawling in the snow. As he sat up, I yelled to ask him if he was okay, and he waved. I took that as a signal that all was well, but then my young son started screaming. When I looked again, I saw blood and watched Andrew slowly slump to the ground.

I slid down the hill as fast as I could. Going into doctor mode, I conducted a quick physical evaluation of his wounds. The stick had sliced across Andrew's forehead, skimming his glasses, then continued down the right side of his face, jaw, and neck. He had deep gashes across his face and neck, with flesh splayed out and blood soaking into the snow. Andrew lay, conscious and moaning, as I kneeled over him, grabbing snow, pushing the gaping wound edges together, and applying hard, cold pressure to his head wounds with both my hands.

The stick had sliced Andrew's scalp and face open with the power of a strong, unyielding razor blade as he rotated around it. His glasses had saved his eyes. I wrapped his head in a turban of scarves, and then we gently carried him out of the basin, slow step by slow step, keeping him conscious and doing our best to stem the bleeding.

Our two-hour trip to the hospital involved a transfer from the first ambulance, which had a limited range of service, to a second one halfway down the mountain. The second rescue team looked at Andrew, his head snuggly wrapped, and seemed to assume we were overreacting to a simple laceration. I was nervous but started second-guessing my own concerns.

Once we reached the emergency room, I had to wash off the blood from my hands and clothes and change into hospital scrubs before being allowed into the emergency room. As I emerged from the hospital bathroom, I heard a trauma code being called. Confused, I realized my husband was no longer in sight. While I had been changing, the nurses had unwrapped his layered scarf bandage and quickly realized he had major lacerations with critical blood loss. They couldn't find a vein to start an IV and his vital signs were unstable, so he was rushed to a trauma room. I found Andrew down the hall, surrounded by a code team who were frantically trying to stabilize his vital signs.

Andrew's wounds went to the very edge of his carotid artery, narrowly missing it. Mercifully, his carotid vein also escaped injury. Many smaller vessels were sliced open, but they were not as critical. A central line inserted into the uninjured side of his neck delivered lifesaving fluids. We were amazed at the power of that little stick—until a doctor explained that the snow is so deep in the basin areas that what look like sticks are actually the tops of large evergreens. Despite massive blood loss and a three-hour surgery to repair layers of tissue, he would heal with only some faint facial scars to tell his story.

Yet during his recovery, he had to face an unseen injury that cut just as deep, if only figuratively. Just prior to the accident, Andrew had been told that his job was being eliminated due to abrupt changes in his firm's leadership. It was a hard loss for him and for our family, as he had previously been assured of rewards, including a future partnership, for his long hours of extra work. However, his employer did make an allowance for a several-month transition period and support through the summer. Partners we had come to know as friends promised to champion him in this difficult time. Several visited him in the hospital and offered words of encouragement and baskets of goodies. Even so, we worried about the time his recovery was taking. Andrew was unsteady, anemic, and jaundiced from all the blood loss into his tissues. He needed to keep working at the firm while also looking for another position.

On the day of his hospital discharge, Andrew's phone rang as I pulled out of the parking lot. His office's managing partner, a trusted colleague, bluntly told Andrew that the firm was terminating his position, effective immediately. It was a simple business decision that had to be made, despite any promises they'd made to him. A new kind of shock set in. And this time, I wasn't able to go into rescue mode. My own fierce anger conflated with Andrew's numbing disorientation.

Andrew was frail for six weeks. His short-term memory was impaired for several months. A quick return to full-time work was no longer possible. Eventually, he began work as a consultant, which allowed him to gradually return to permanent work in a new position. But despite physical healing, he remained bloodied in the basin emotionally, disoriented and unable to get to higher ground. He had trusted appearances that camouflaged cover-ups. The climb out was prolonged, arduous, and fearful.

As the months wore on after the accident and job loss, the external wounds became harder to notice. But it felt as if we were in a slow-moving ambulance with a crew giving rote reassurances while the bleeding continued under wraps. I wanted to probe the injury and still felt the closeness of betrayal. Andrew remained incredulous at the firm's actions, but he didn't speak at all about his near-death experience. We survived that time, but the repercussions of the wound afflicted us for years.

◌

Wounds are a universal human experience. From scraped knees to torn ligaments to life-threatening lacerations like Andrew's, our bodies become injured through both use and disuse, through unintentional and sometimes very intentional means. Wounds may be self-inflicted or inflicted by another person, animal, or object. We even blame God for some wounds—at least on insurance forms—such as when lightning strikes. Occasionally, we actually choose to be wounded, knowing it is a necessary route to ultimate healing—surgical procedures are typically undertaken for this reason.

Most of us live our lives with no idea of the complexity of the wound-healing process. Just as we take for granted the regular beating of our heart, we simply count on healing to be there for us, always ready and always in top shape. The importance of healthy wound healing, not just on an individual level, but also on a societal one, is enormous. Over 6.5 million people in the United States have a chronic wound that won't heal.[1] Caring for acute wounds also imposes an enormous demand on health care—wound care after surgery, wound infections, and wound scarring are major problems. A modest estimate of the amount spent on wound care is $31 billion annually.[2] Getting wound healing right, as fully and efficiently as possible, is a major goal of the medical and scientific community.

Fortunately, our body's wound-healing system does seem to work almost flawlessly most of the time. It certainly is elegant, as are so many of the subprocesses we are coming to understand as we go deeper into the mystery of the human body. The healing phases are precise, interdependent, and directed toward wholeness.

The four overlapping but distinct stages of wound healing are the central images of this book, which we will turn to again and again. The first stage is *hemostasis*, or clotting. Then *inflammation*, an important defensive posture that brings in critical helping cells, follows. New *tissue formation* and maturation develop next. Finally, *remodeling* occurs, which is key to future function and restoration of health. Usually remodeling leads to some scar tissue, but discoveries such as those made in Bem's work may help advance tissue regeneration and full restoration of new tissue, known as scar-free healing.

FOUR STAGES OF WOUND HEALING

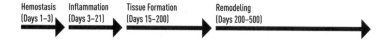

Clotting, inflammation, tissue formation, and remodeling serve as our signposts in wound healing. If the separate critical stages are interrupted or don't follow the proper order, things go predictably off course. Self-injury, infection, harmful growths, and inflexible scars are a few outcomes that can occur from impaired wound healing.

Other problems may occur in bodies that don't adequately feel pain. Hansen's disease (formerly called leprosy) and diabetes, for instance, cause neuropathies in which pain sensors in the body are dulled. With these diseases, wounds may actually fester and become worse, because when the body can't signal pain, the injuries aren't as easily recognized. But even people with intact nervous systems don't immediately recognize the pain of a serious wound like a bullet as their body first tries to protect them in a shock-like state.

Hidden unhealed wounds have a way of becoming visible. In medicine, we sometimes see inflammation grow until a deep abscess breaks open—a burst appendix is a common example. Leftover debris in wound sites presents a particular problem. At first, the body tries to wall it off, to encapsulate it. But the longer it goes unrecognized, the greater the chance for an infection to develop. Sometimes, leftover debris in a puncture wound site will work its way to the skin surface as the skin forms new layers from below. Pieces of glass, splinters of wood, and stitches have found their way up and out like this. Unhealed wounds can also form tunnels, called sinus tracts. These tunnels hide the wound origins but drain infection into an open space, like the mouth or neck. The surgeon has to follow the tunnel to its source rather than simply close the opening, or it will never heal.

Similarly, our hidden unhealed wounds of the spirit will make themselves known, causing people to leave their spouse, their church, and their longtime friends. Withdrawal, anger, and self-destructive habits can occur when healing doesn't. The tragedies of post-traumatic stress disorder and suicide are dramatic results of earlier unhealed trauma. In American society, and especially in our churches, people increasingly seem to separate themselves into encapsulated defensive groups rather than resolve to clear the debris and seek closure. We avoid conflicting viewpoints instead of working together to heal wounds that cause division. Separation is not a sign of health.

Polarization in America is at an all-time high, not just politically but also socially. For example, mainline Protestant churches used to have members who might be described as theologically conservative, moderate, or liberal, all worshiping together. Perhaps tradition drove attendance, but in any case, a spectrum of views was clearly present within these large denominations. Now, though, individual churches tend to draw people who are like-minded, with little room for those who hold different ways of thinking. Congregations are becoming less diverse, following the same patterns as political and social movements, abandoning any uniting middle ground. Dan White Jr. laments this in his book *Love over Fear*, challenging Christians to see polarization as a force that destroys community and ultimately tears apart the kingdom of God. White cites Pew research that shows a "siloing" effect: 73 percent of self-described conservatives say that their close friends share their same worldview, and similarly 69 percent of those claiming a liberal leaning.[3]

Experts in church demographics show these changes visually. What was formerly a bell curve distribution of shared beliefs among members is now inverted, with two peaks on the far extremes and a long shallow space in the middle. This inverse curve depicting polarization looks like a deep gaping wound, impossible to close without a graft.

POLARIZATION OF CHURCH BELIEFS

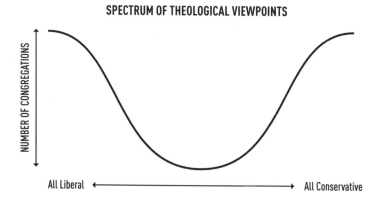

SPECTRUM OF THEOLOGICAL VIEWPOINTS

NUMBER OF CONGREGATIONS

All Liberal ⟵⟶ All Conservative

Recently, our deeply hurtful wounds have found a different way to surface—through social media. Hashtags with galvanizing phrases gain thousands of shares and personal comments. Triggered by public events, people disclose their secrets to a faceless world before revealing them to their closest family members. To many, it may seem safer to share our stories of assault, discrimination, or feuds on a screen than in a pew or in a dining room. We receive acceptance, encouragement, and even words of love from people we may never meet in person. Paradoxically, we use that same media to hurt those we know well by unfriending or hiding posts from neighbors with whom we disagree or by "ghosting" a romantic partner as a way to end our relationship.

Of course, not all of our personal wounds are deep and life-threatening. Some are like a childhood scraped knee. We get a cute Band-Aid and move on, ignoring it after a day or two. A few minor disagreements with a partner or a pastor rarely cause a split. But an inability to recognize and voice disagreement, to go through the stages necessary for restoration of relational trust and communication, does lead to isolation, a walling off, and an eventual rupture with scarring. The accumulation of such scars can become crippling over time.

Businesses understand that wound prevention is critical to their prosperity. They promote healthy workplaces and avoid divisive corporate lesions. Not long ago, many organizational leaders encouraged us to think of the workplace as a family. I never embraced this metaphor, wanting to maintain a clear separation between the roles of family and work. Now workplaces have moved on to other conceptual models, many using the idea of teams, hiring well-paid consultant coaches to help them succeed as winning organizations. I guess a consultant coach is better than a consultant mama!

Another group embraces their conceptual identity as a family, and has done so for two thousand years. As brothers and sisters of Jesus, and sons and daughters of the Father, this family is mysteriously knit together and fundamentally inseparable through time and space. The church—the collection of Christians worldwide—is also called the body of Christ: one body with many members.[4] The idea echoes what scientists are also affirming: that the universe acts as an organism, with every part of it related and interdependent upon the whole. Whether it is the threat of a pandemic like COVID-19, the global climate change that affects individual places in a variety of ways, or the solar system's patterns of moons circling planets, the pull of one body on another—one element affecting many others—is becoming more apparent. Understanding ourselves as members of one body is a powerful image that can be understood anew as we examine how wounds heal in both scientific and metaphorical terms.

If the church is meant to mirror the body, with all of its amazing powers to heal from wounds, why is it split into so many pieces? There have been schisms since early Christianity, deep gashes that separated the faithful from one another as disputes about both doctrine and practice ruptured the community. Throughout the centuries, the separations have continued, as denominational and cultural understandings limit fellowship at the Communion table and beyond. Even within individual churches, steady streams of people move in and out of membership, often due to unhealed wounds. Reconciliation may appear too difficult, even hopeless, and this loss of hope is a fatal blow to the Christian body.

Part of the problem may be in the idea of "church" as an organization rather than an organism, though the latter is certainly implied by the term *the body of Christ*. We are a gathering of individual people in a particular place, but we are also mystically united. Communion, in the double sense of that word, marks the body of Christ as both Eucharist and gathered members. Wound healing at the personal, group, societal, and body of Christ level is an *organic* process more than an organizational one, depending upon a dynamic interrelationship of living beings who are constantly changing, maturing, growing, dying, and starting over. In that process, *all* are changed—the wounded and the community in relationship with them.

The human body's natural wound-healing system provides analogies as we seek ways to mirror those processes while we strive to heal our social wounds. In some ways, we have always borrowed from the terminology of the body's wound response in discussing our emotional and group wounds.

- She is scarred.
- He is raw.
- They are sensitive.

- This organization is a bloody mess.
- The leadership is too inflamed to think rationally.
- Our friendship is ruptured.
- Her marriage is broken.
- Someone needs to stop the bleeding in that church since the pastor left!

The problem is, our language betrays a dependence on terminology related to crisis management and wounds that don't heal rather than words that portray a slow collaborative movement toward health.

Bem turns this familiar language use on its head as she describes the incredibly intricate process of biological wound healing at the molecular and genetic level. Rather than relying on a disorganized, individual, and crisis-oriented response, Bem sees how the body is created with a framework that promotes full restoration and regeneration. As she works to develop new therapies for wound healing based on discoveries in molecular genetics, she is immersed in a hidden world, a place she calls her secret garden, where collaboration and community are central to success, where all the individual components are crucial to the task of repair, and where diversity is necessary for a unified whole to emerge.

As Bem teaches spiritual leaders to appreciate science as a friend to faith, she illustrates how our bodies don't react to physical wounds merely with emergency responses or limiting quick fixes. The actual healing process is complex, involving distinct stages and many cell types contributing to the overall work in an orderly, patient progression. There is some variation by individual characteristics, such as age and immune status, but enough consistency to count upon it as an incredibly reliable system. Scientists still haven't fully mined its depths but routinely refer to it with words that speak of its art as much as its chemical compositions. Wound healing is described as *beautiful* and *choreographed*. Some compare it to a symphony orchestra, an apt description since, all along the way, there are section leaders, sequential movements, rare soloists, stage crew, patrons, publicists, mediators, set designers, and conductors. New works emerge from the collective performance.

Through these four separate stages, wounds are replaced by new structures—blood vessels, skin, and nerves—a truly transformational process. At times, scarring is the best that can be accomplished to close the wound. Not all wounds are survivable. But as we look at how the body is designed to react, we can see a realm of possibilities that offer integration, diversity, support, beauty, and possibility to our own hidden wounds.

As we compare and contrast our physical and nonphysical wounds, terminology is important. Are we talking about emotional wounds? Spiritual? Psychological? Relational seems like an apt descriptor, but perhaps the truest word is *corporate*. That word can conjure up big business, but its Latin root is *corpus*, meaning "in the form of a body." A corporation is simply a group of people united as one body for a common purpose. And so the wounds we will consider with fresh eyes are really our corporate ones—those affecting our joined relationships with one another, whether in the family, society, or houses of worship. Their effects are shared, and their healing requires community.

To illustrate this, we begin with the story of a boy, a dart, and a clot.

CHAPTER 2

FRESHLY INJURED

Stop the Bleeding and Keep Things Clean

*A Samaritan traveling the road came on him. When he
saw the man's condition, his heart went out to him. He gave
him first aid, disinfecting and bandaging his wounds.*

LUKE 10:33-34, MSG

NEAR THE END of a long, boring Saturday night in the pediatric emergency department where I served my residency, the medics rolled a young teen into the trauma area. I glanced up, then stared. The boy on the stretcher had a large silver dart coming out of the left side of his head. He appeared perfectly stable, alert, and embarrassed. He was also glaring at an older boy, who was standing next to him. As the two began arguing, it became apparent that they were brothers. The older one had thrown the dart, but it wasn't clear whether he'd hurled the stray throw on a dare or intentionally, or whether he simply had horrible aim. The story was muddled, as stories told by fighting siblings—one with a dart in his skull—are apt to be.

In his fury, the younger boy hadn't let anyone in his family touch him, which turned out to be a good thing. The neurosurgeons needed to see where the tip of the dart was before removing it. Infection and bleeding risk depended on how deeply it went. So William Tell, as he became known to one and all that night, was wheeled through the basement hospital corridors to the CT scanner with a dart in his head. The wonderful news was that the dart had just missed hitting the lining of his brain, so surgeons could safely pull it out. All he had to deal with was a little bleeding, some mild swelling, and a new nickname.

The tissue destruction was limited to the diameter and length of the dart. Since it didn't strike any major blood vessels, his bleeding was due to tears in the walls of small capillaries, easily patched by the body's hemostasis team. The body's inflammation crew cleared the area of any foreign cells, although the surgeons took care to do that as well. William Tell's body successfully completed the first phase of healing, the only one needed to address his wound.

The instant an injury occurs, pain receptors located in the walls of blood vessels trigger the body's reaction. Hemostasis, which literally means to stop bleeding, is the body's first response to a wound—and a logical one. No committee meetings, no consensus building; just an urgent command to stop the flow of blood. The very second the wall of a blood vessel is wounded, the blood vessel spasms and constricts, automatically limiting blood flow out of the injured vessel. Platelets, cell fragments that act like pieces of Velcro, then begin sticking to the injured area of the vessel wall, starting the formation of a clot. Fortunately for William Tell, hemostasis begins within ten seconds of an injury, whether it be a dart to the head or a brother's black eye.

Through the release of enzymes, platelets call for more platelets as they start sticking to the site of the wound. Fibrin strands begin to form a mesh, similar to a gauze pad, for the platelets to stick to, making a base for the developing clot. Only one minute has passed since the injury.

With the fibrin mesh in place, signals are sent from the enzymes so that the blood goes from liquid to gel—it coagulates. The platelets and blood cells in the wound area then form a plug in the hole until new tissue can grow or a new vessel can sprout to take the injured one's place. We don't bleed out from every pin prick, razor cut, or whack on the head because of the quick action of our platelets and coagulation mechanisms, which allow the blood to adapt its form at the site of the wound.

William Tell's wound didn't need much of an inflammatory response. But in cases of major trauma, inflammation is recognized as critically tied in with hemostasis. They are two sides of the same coin, each responsive to the other. The moment the blood vessel wall is injured, it reacts with both a hemostatic response and an inflammatory one. The first inflammatory action is the leaking of a fluid, called a transudate, into the tissues surrounding the injured blood vessel wall. Transudate, which is made of water, salt, and protein, makes the tissue swell. Like a pressure bandage, the swelling helps control bleeding and also helps prevent infection at the wound site.

Meanwhile, the platelets activated in hemostasis not only form a sticky clot, but also help call and capture cells like neutrophils and monocytes. These are part of the body's white blood cell system and are designated as inflammatory cells. They fight infection by eating bacteria, sending out enzymes that destroy foreign cells, and swallowing up dead and fragmented debris at the wound site. The white blood cells get caught up in transudate too, and they stay in the area like an infantry of soldiers to defend the wound from further deterioration.

We've changed the way we treat people with major trauma and life-threatening infections as we have grown to better understand the ways hemostasis and inflammation work together in stabilizing an assault to the body. We used to see them as very separate occurrences, with hemostasis important to countering trauma and inflammation important in controlling infection. Now we see them as twin events, inextricably linked together. We treat people as if they have both issues—trauma and infection—even if what we believe is happening is primarily blood loss or primarily an infectious-disease process.

In this first defensive phase of wound healing, the body takes immediate action—not a second is lost. This phase, so urgently assembled and functional, lessens the impact of both minor and serious wounds. When staged properly, it stabilizes the situation until more definitive repair can take place.

Bickering between brothers, however, may take more time to resolve.

CR

In what ways can the initial response to the wounds in our corporate lives mimic those in our physical bodies? If our analogy holds, defense is meant for rapid stabilization, a first phase on the way toward ultimate healing.

In 1996, Bem had just finished years of graduate school, attaining her doctorate while her husband also had a bright career in technological sciences. Then everything changed overnight. Julio was diagnosed with a rare, incurable bone marrow disease called polycythemia, which creates an over-production of red blood cells. The opposite of anemia, poly-cythemia causes the blood to become so thick and sludge-like that the treatment is to bleed the patient in order to prevent strokes and clots.

At first, Bem and Julio operated as if on autopilot, rapidly rearranging their schedules because of Julio's exhaustion and frequent treatments. Then Bem found out she was preg-nant. Not long after she and Julio had been broadsided by his illness, she was put on strict bed rest for the first tri-mester.

During traumatic life events, our physical bodies do activate a type of biological defense that helps us navigate the initial moments following devastating news. Our brains don't let the enormity of the situation sink in, numbing us to the reality so that we can promptly take action in a sort of suspended shock-like state. That's what kept Bem and Julio functioning in the days immediately following Julio's diagnosis and word of Bem's pregnancy. In any such emergency, it's almost as if there is some clotting and coagulation of the emotions—we make it through receiving a devastating diagnosis, planning a funeral, or being told that our child is ill or our house is destroyed. We wait until the flow of urgent issues has slowed a bit before we take a look at how deep the wound is.

After that, outside support can play a crucial role. Once their health was at risk and their work schedules were upended, logic told Julio and Bem that it was time to end their American sojourn, despite the clear sense of vocation that had initiated it, and return to their families in the Philippines. When Bem told her closest friend that she and Julio needed to leave Tennessee, her friend responded by immediately organizing a coalition of church members to show them that family was also present in that time and place, and this family could sustain them through the crisis. Back in the Philippines, Bem's sister was skeptical. "Are you sure these Americans can care for you the way we do here? I hear that they value independence and privacy. Are you sure you don't want to come home?"

For Bem, broccoli-chicken casserole came to symbolize the adhesive grip of platelets joining platelets in a great clump, eventually forming a plug in a fearful wound. She recalls:

*For many months our friends came to clean our house,
do our laundry, and mow our yard. They also brought
a steady stream of food—satisfying chicken-broccoli
casseroles, warm crusty corn bread, soft green beans,
flaky biscuits with butter and honey, sweet apple
dumplings, and chicken noodle soup. Those casseroles
gave me great joy—and I don't even like broccoli.
I didn't even know what a casserole was when we
immigrated to the USA twenty-eight years ago! In
my birth country, the Philippines, electricity is very
expensive and only the wealthy can afford modern
ovens. But here in Tennessee and the South, casseroles
are ubiquitous, especially when tragedy strikes. My
husband and I ate a lot of Southern comfort food
when our lives were turned upside down.*

*We were so stunned and scared. Like a blood clot,
these interwoven coordinated acts of kindness helped
stop the overwhelming flood of fear and anxiety, and
provided some needed stability and provisional structure
as we slowly regained our bearings and adapted to the
radical changes in our lives—frequent visits to clinics
and hospitals, caring for a baby boy, and finding new
jobs that accommodated our challenging schedules.*

Sometimes, depending upon our cultural and family
experiences, we've been taught to avoid acknowledging the
wounds of even close friends and relatives. We take a slow
approach and write a card or wait for the hurt one to bring it

up before we say anything. But if the body reacted this way, we'd have an oozing wound, one that took longer to heal, with more infection and bleeding.

It can be difficult to know if it is our role to be on the first line of defense. It does take discernment to know when to intervene. The closer we are to the hurt—whether we or a loved one are experiencing it—the more clearly we are touched by that injury. Does the pain cause us to constrict? Fear often feels constricting. But if we constrict when faced with a corporate wound, it may signal that we are to act like the blood vessel, where constricting is a positive message that signals help is needed. Are we part of the first line of defense? Withdrawal would not be the right response then, even if we feel ourselves tightening up. We may feel we don't know what to do, but a complex solution is not required at this point. Rapid defense just requires a recognition of the situation and a willingness to help stem the bleeding by leaning in closely. Sometimes the best quick response is just a simple affirmation of how sad and difficult the situation is.

Acknowledging a wound and its severity can be lifesaving. Conversely, denying them can be deadly. We sometimes hide our wounds because we are embarrassed, think we deserved or caused the problem, or fear the consequences if others see the injury. When I was in college many years ago, all three reasons were in play when my friend, who also happened to be well-known as a campus leader, was being physically abused by her fiancé. We tried to support her but didn't know how to make a difference. None of us had seen public information about domestic violence back then, and whenever we tried to speak directly to her about our concern for her, she responded with shame and guilt. Wanting to spare her further pain, we backed off.

Perhaps worse than self-denial is when a revelation of hurt is responded to with doubt rather than affirmation. Those who courageously share about their wounds to someone they hope they can trust need to hear "I believe you!" followed by "I will help you" or "How can I help you?" These are critical responses for someone freshly wounded. They can help stem the bleeding.

Responding to repetitive wounds is particularly difficult. The wounded and their supporters alike can become fatigued as time goes on, both from failed past efforts to heal and a weakening of overall defense systems. In my own life, I experienced persistent wounding by a close family member. This frightening, unpredictable, and deeply injurious relationship existed for years. Throughout childhood and into my early adulthood, well-meaning folks typically responded to me in one of two ways. They either dismissed my pain by saying, "The person doesn't mean it" and "Don't let it bother you," or they asked, "Why is this happening? What do you do to incite it?" Those responses failed to shore me up, to slow the bleeding, and to clear the debris so I could move forward in healing.

Finally, one person witnessed another painful interaction and quietly remarked: "That is so sad; I'm really sorry." A rush of emotion filled me, and I carried a lighter spirit for its having been acknowledged. His words served as a clot, plugging this fresh wound.

FIRST RESPONDERS

In this first phase of healing corporate wounds, quick action and a healthy defense system are needed. This is not the time for arguing about fault lines, assigning blame, or going into panic mode. We need to stop the bleeding at its site. Keep focused on the wound at hand, not past ones. Form a clot. Clean up the debris. Gather around with positive pressure. Then be ready to get out of the way when things stabilize if we aren't the best people for the next phase. Everyone has a role, but everyone doesn't have every role. How do we discern ours?

Rehearse rapid but measured defensive responses

If we haven't practiced reacting well to little incidents—the equivalent of William Tell's dart—we will be unable to do so when a major crisis hits. Developmentally, the easiest time to learn and practice these responses is when we are quite young. I called one technique that I used with my children "replay." When the children behaved badly, such as when one impatiently grabbed a toy and another called that sibling a name, I made them do another take of their interaction. We pretended we were on a movie set and had to reshoot the scene. Sometimes it took a while, with me as director calling, "Cut!" and starting it all again. We ran through such episodes until we got them right—even the angriest siblings eventually spoke to each other kindly in order to end the exercise!

I've passed this technique on to some of my patients' families, helping their children cope with their anger not with spitting, kicking, or slamming doors, but with words, gentleness, and respect. Practicing a behavior is the only way to truly learn it. The trick is learning how to safely practice a new defense system when we are adults.

Generally, we assume most defensive systems are big and strong, like linebackers or army tanks, using power and intimidation to overcome the opponent. Our bodies have something to teach us here as well. If they mounted such a mighty response when we were wounded, our platelets would be too bulky to get to the site, and we wouldn't have such a large reserve of interacting components rapidly moving from one place to the next. The transudate has to squeeze out into the extracellular tissue space, the platelets have to adhere against the vessel wall, and the inflammatory cells have to wrap around debris. The blood changes shape as it coagulates. All these parts are nimble, flexible, and adaptable to the situation. I wonder how many interpersonal conflicts would heal more swiftly if, instead of reacting quickly with a defensive show of power, anger, and righteousness, we instead rapidly sought to tamp down the hurt, bend toward the other, and surrender some of our own agenda? I know I would have avoided a number of prolonged difficulties had I reacted that way. The writer of Proverbs understood this: "A gentle answer turns away wrath, but a harsh word stirs up anger" (Proverbs 15:1, NIV).

Cultivate contemplative prayer

One practice we may cultivate to improve our rapid defense system is contemplative prayer. It has a long tradition in the Eastern Orthodox and Roman Catholic church, but the Protestant world and nonchurched folks may be less familiar with it. Thomas Keating, Thomas Merton, Dallas Willard, and Richard Rohr are four contemporary Christian writers whose materials are accessible for anyone with an interest in this practice. Essentially, praying in this reflective, deliberate way involves purposeful stillness, active listening, humble receiving, and ultimate enjoyment of the presence of God. Ironically, learning to slow down and listen can prepare us to quickly bring calm and wisdom when a wound occurs.

When the world was overtaken by COVID-19, we were all hurtled into a time of uncertainty coupled with relentless commentary on what was unfolding. One day's understanding unraveled the next day. As a health-care provider, I was swept up in the onslaught of information and asked to provide commentary as well as hands-on relief. At first, I found myself glued to multiple news outlets and constantly distracted, having difficulty paying attention to anything that required sustained thought.

But returning to intentional periods of contemplative prayer each day began centering me in stillness so I could turn more fully to the day ahead. It is a practice I continue. I also use the Pray as You Go app, as it gives a daily reading, meditation, music, and prayer.[1] Sometimes all it takes is to sit quietly for five minutes, asking God to help me be aware of his presence. Keating shows us how to do centering prayer by breathing in and out while focusing on one aspect of God, such as his trustworthiness, love, or mercy.

Others are drawn to meditation. There are numerous apps for that, as well. One practice that helped me in the midst of the pandemic is termed *RAIN*:

Recognize what is happening
Allow the experience
Investigate it gently
Nurture the wounded spot[2]

This guided meditation is designed to help us come to terms with what is happening and give compassion to ourselves and others.

Being able to still ourselves in the midst of the urgent noise of our world, especially when chaos clamors for a personal emotional response, is a critical skill that takes time and discipline yet yields peace in times of suffering and controversy. And peace, said the apostle Paul, is what we are called to as members of one body (Colossians 3:15).

Engage in intercessory prayer
Prayer is bidirectional, or more rightly, multidirectional. Like the enzymes that call out for help, it signals a message from the wounded or their helpers to an unseen point, expecting a response that defies the limits of time and space. The

responses come in many forms, not all known, some just right for starting a clot. Perhaps the more practical among us could practice rapid response prayer more regularly, those fast intercessory prayers that ask for God's will to be done and for wisdom to understand what that is.

Clear the clutter

The role of inflammation is a curious one. It sounds so negative. To call another person *inflammatory* is certainly not a compliment. But in the context of a healthy defense system, inflammation plays a positive role—engaging the immune system to ward off infection and keep the injured area clean. In the case of a corporate wound, rather than being seen as inflammatory personalities, the people playing this role can be viewed as sweepers—cleaning up messes behind the scenes. They are like the stage crew on a movie set, arranging everything for the best take and removing articles that don't belong in that particular shot.

Faith communities were asked to stop gathering as the pandemic spread. Some met that request with resistance. How would people without technology access remote services? What did fellowship, faith, and trust look like when everyone was separate and secluded? But most congregations quickly complied, providing a rapid defense during the crushing times.

Helpers with expertise in technology assisted others so they could join platforms like Zoom. Facebook groups started to pop up, offering access not just to members of local faith communities, but to anyone who wanted to participate. Professional musicians like Yo-Yo Ma and Itzhak Perlman offered free virtual concerts—even online lessons. Clots were starting to form in the gaping wound that seemed to have no edges.

More and more ways of standing in unity emerged from this initial loss. My own church offered a daily prayer service over Facebook. My small group gathered every Friday by teleconference to support and encourage each other, and our attendance actually increased in this newfound state. People shared through social media how they were managing to control their tempers and find new ways to constructively deal with the tensions of being cooped up. And humor helped, from the late-night talk show host who showed his vulnerability when performing in front of his children to the "work at home" memes that circulated. As we stuck together, avoided criticism, and cleaned up what we could in the pandemic's destruction, we saw healing take shape in new ways.

Offer tangible support

Bem had seen such first-line defense long before the COVID-19 crisis. One of the most wounding typhoons of all time—Super Typhoon Yolanda—tore through the Philippines in 2013. Filipinos are used to recurrent typhoons. Neighbors try to save one another during floods, and private individuals load their trucks, cars, or vans with groceries and head to the areas affected. Churches and schools become evacuation shelters and centers for distribution of food.

Traditionally, the first to respond from abroad to calamity in the Philippines are fellow Filipinos. They send money and pack relief goods to mail in what are called balikbayan boxes (named after the Tagalog word for a returning Filipino), which they know will reach personal homes and churches before any official aid can be gathered and organized. Their quick organized actions give a lifeline when every moment is critical, rapidly forming a clot to stem the bleeding.

Yet Typhoon Yolanda was far more devastating than other storms, killing more than seven thousand people in that island nation alone, leaving more than 1.9 million homeless and more than six million displaced.[3] Many small island areas were impassable, the infrastructure was completely wiped out, and the most urgent task was getting water and food, as well as medical and sanitary supplies, to remote islands. These areas were accessible only via dangerous land travel through guerilla gang–controlled territories, or by air travel sponsored by international charities that were at odds with the government's policies and considered a threat to the leaders' power.

Corruption and politics could have delayed the desperately needed relief. But instead, international aid agencies creatively and quickly collaborated to secure an entire uninhabited island in the region and turn it into an aid station and field hospital. Political alliances were temporarily suspended and a route was set up for air transport of those needing the most immediate medical care, as well as for planes bringing in relief supplies. That island of safety became the first fibrin mesh clot to form for many who had lost hope.

I've seen other examples closer to home of people joining together to save others. A few years ago, I saw a news report showing truckers parked in both directions under a highway overpass. The strange picture was the result of police shutting down the interstate and then asking thirteen nearby truckers to drive their rigs to the site of a life-threatening event. A man was on the overpass, contemplating suicide by jumping off the railing onto the highway. Like sticky platelets, the trucks lined up, one next to the other, and provided a barrier between the man and the concrete below. After a few hours, police convinced the man to leave the overpass and get help.[4]

The defensive reaction is like that—immediate, in the right place at the right time, and then gone as fast as it began. It does not seek to patch everything up immediately, as we sometimes try to do when we give advice or ask questions as a loved one's crisis is unfolding. What is really needed in those first moments is someone to come alongside to stop the bleeding, stick with the situation, and be a platelet that clots and then activates others to offer help. As we've discussed, individuals function pretty well in the immediate moments of a crisis, but that does not mean folks are actually thinking well, able to make nonurgent decisions or handle everything themselves. They function due to the gift of shock, which is limited to the very immediate details of what they must endure.

CR

Stop the bleeding and keep it clean. It seems so simple. Yet life shows us over and over that the simple rules are the hardest to live by. Our initial responses to corporate injury, whether the injury is intentional or unintentional, momentary or life-threatening, are often rapid and instinctual but may not align with processes that stabilize and offer the healthiest routes to full recovery.

May our imaginations be inspired as we consider how we can stick close to the side of a hurting friend, swiftly calling in others for reinforcements to help stabilize the scene. We can then apply positive pressure with kindness, our peaceful presence, and lawnmowers and casseroles. Painful ill-timed advice, suggestions about blame, or platitudes on the ultimate meaning of pain and loss have no place among first responders. And for those of us who have ever been called inflammatory, we can laugh as we remember that in conflicts, inflammation helps rid the body of what hinders healing and keeps the site as pure as possible.

CHAPTER 3

INFLAMMATION GONE AWRY
Slow Boils and Explosive Storms

They have healed the wound of my people lightly, saying,
"Peace, peace," when there is no peace.

JEREMIAH 8:11

MOLOKAI IS BEST KNOWN as the Hawaiian island where people
with leprosy were exiled between the 1860s and the 1960s.
Though the illness is properly termed Hansen's disease, the
local residents still refer to it as leprosy, and a US Public
Health Service facility remains active on the flat volcanic
peninsula that stretches away from the base of some of the
highest sea cliffs in the world. Only those sixteen and older
are allowed to visit this area, and only with a registered host.
This isn't due to fears of contagion but to protect the privacy
of the handful of elderly residents who call the site home after
a lifetime of inhabiting this tiny spot in the Pacific.[1]

Hansen's disease is treatable, and contagion may be

47

arrested by early drug treatment—much like the treatment for tuberculosis (TB). It isn't nearly as easy to get infected with Hansen's as it is to get TB or the flu. In fact, only about 5 percent of the world's population is readily susceptible to it.[2] The Hawaiian people seem particularly genetically susceptible to the strain that sent thousands to permanent exile on Molokai. The stigma, though, is still overwhelming, which discourages people from seeking treatment.

Hansen's disease brings up several common images for those who have never seen the disease. Most people think of characters in biblical stories, of outcasts considered unclean and with disfiguring deformities. There is some debate as to whether biblical leprosy was the same disease as the current illness, but we do know that the type of Hansen's disease in India today has been there for at least four thousand years. As such an ancient disease, it has shaped many cultural responses to illness, contagion, and healing.

While the term *leprosy* has induced fear across the centuries, the real culprit behind much of the scourge is not the bacteria known as *Mycobacterium leprae*, but our body's immune reaction to it. An infection with *M. leprae* sets off a series of inflammatory responses that are never resolved. Rather, the inflammation grows and grows, stuck in a self-perpetuating cycle. Looking more closely at Hansen's as well as at diseases like cancer and COVID-19, we can see what havoc is wrought by an inflammatory response that is too intense for the situation at hand.

I've worked in several places where Hansen's disease is

still present: Molokai, India, the Dominican Republic, and Micronesia. While hundreds of patients came to the weekly clinics we held in India back in 1985, most of the cases I've seen since then have been in elderly patients dealing with long-term effects of their infections. In the summer of 2018, I visited a public health center on an island in Micronesia, which, like Hawaii, has a long history of dealing with this disease. On the wall of the clinic, I saw bright posters that depicted early warning signs on the skin—flat numb patches that are lighter than the surrounding skin—with messages that encouraged people to speak up if they had any signs of leprosy.

I noticed another wall with very different posters. These depicted the long-term results of neglecting early treatment of specific illnesses. One showed the devastation of progressive leprous lesions; another showed diabetic leg and foot ulcers. Frankly, they were nothing you would want to look at, but the tiny, cramped room made it unavoidable. The posters featured full-color photographs of legs and feet covered with purple and red, open, oozing sores. Blackened toes and heels deformed by chronic ulcers and tissue loss showed late effects of disease. Those who couldn't read wouldn't know the posters were showing different diseases—diabetes and Hansen's—as the lesions looked so similar.

On the top of a file cabinet in the same crowded clinic was a plastic model of a foot with conspicuous, deeply set, bright red ulcers. The clinic doctor was trying, through every means possible, to prevent complications of both ancient tropical and modern chronic diseases. Though Hansen's disease was only a mild threat, the incidence of diabetes was exploding. This island had the highest rate in Micronesia and double that on the mainland United States. Sadly, the islanders were trading their sustainable diet of taro, fish, crab, and fresh fruit for soda, Spam, pizza, burgers, and alcohol.

Some of the most serious, complex, and chronic effects of both Hansen's disease and diabetes are caused indirectly. When left unchecked and poorly controlled, both diseases lead to complications that, once initiated, become incredibly frustrating to manage and undo. Chronic inflammation with ulcers is one of those effects. Those ulcers are truly ugly; they often teem with bacteria and have a putrid smell. Despite daily dressing changes, debridement (scraping away the dead tissue and cleaning the area), antibiotics, and careful attempts to avoid pressure on the tissue, many ulcers continue to fester. Amputations and sepsis (deadly blood infections) are common consequences of persistently nonhealing ulcers.

Neuropathy is a cardinal feature of Hansen's disease—all those skin patches are numb, and the numbness ends up extending to the fingers, feet, nose, and face. When people can't feel pain, they may not realize they have an injury, such as a splinter or a small cut. Left untreated, these minor wounds become infected and burgeon into abscesses or ulcers that won't heal. This is such a serious problem in Hansen's disease that when I worked in India, the hospital employed a full-time sandal maker who fashioned tailor-made shoes for patients so their foot ulcers would be kept from pressure points.

Diabetes also leads to neuropathy, which is due to glucose damage at the cellular level and blood flow damage to the tissues. Tiny vessels become clogged when blood sugar is elevated and the tissues don't get enough oxygen-filled blood delivered to them. Numbness and poor blood flow to the feet and lower legs cause what most people simply term poor circulation. As the blood travels from the heart through the blood vessels to organs and limbs, it carries insufficient oxygen, a condition known as hypoxia. As a result, microinfarcts—tiny tissue deaths—occur. Fluids pool and stagnate rather than move. Transudates, the liquids that cause soft tissues to swell following an injury, overdo it, leaking into good tissue. Stationary swelling causes pressure on even more of the surrounding tissues, making things progressively worse. Tissues keep dying from this pressure and the lack of blood and oxygen. They collapse, like a sinkhole, into an ulcerative mess at the sites where the circulation is cut off.

So my doctor friend in Micronesia was right to focus on prevention of these difficult-to-heal situations. I don't know if the scary posters work in his culture. I'm not sure they do in mine. Diabetes in the United States is largely the result of a sedentary lifestyle and poor diet. Knowing these facts, however, rarely changes behavior in our culture; instead, instant gratification usually wins out over slow, incremental change.

In addition to causing local problems like skin ulcers, the inflammatory response can go rogue in a widespread manner throughout the whole body. This happens in cancers, in autoimmune diseases, and in diseases such as COVID-19, which is responsible for the devastating pandemic that began in early 2020. Most people recover from a COVID-19 infection with only mild symptoms. In these cases, the body's immune response is well-matched to the threatening virus. A proper amount of inflammation occurs, causing a fever and maybe some tissue swelling and a cough from the body's infection-fighting cells that are globbed up with the viral particles in the throat. But in a smaller number of cases, people experience overwhelming illness. Their sudden deterioration is sometimes due to the viral load—the number of viral particles that have replicated—becoming massive and damaging the lung tissue. But more often, it is due to the body's own immune reaction, one that propels an inflammatory reaction on a scale that cannot be kept in check.

When the COVID-19 virus triggers a hyperinflammatory response, the body sets off a disordered reaction rather than a controlled inflammatory response. Under ordinary circumstances, neutrophils, commonly called white blood cells, surround invading germs and signal the release of a number of other cell mediators to help swallow up, kill, and dispose of the hostile foreign particles. But in hyperinflammation, huge numbers of neutrophils are released by the body, and they keep sending out destructive enzymes called cytokines.[3] A cytokine storm results.

Cytokines are enzymes that dissolve or break apart proteins, like muscle. When limited, cytokines destroy only the debris from the virus. They may cause some local damage if put out in excess over an extended period of time, like the ulcers caused by too many digestive enzymes. But in a cytokine storm, they can damage good tissue on a massive scale. A large number of immune fighters join in with the cytokines, destroying lung tissue and causing widespread destruction to the body's other vital organs, creating a crisis from which it is almost impossible to recover.

When the cytokines overproduce, either slowly as in chronic inflammation or more catastrophically as in the storms associated with COVID-19, they not only cause tissue deterioration, but they also leave a lot of local debris. The repeated tissue damage signals the inflammation cycle to continue, so it is self-perpetuating. The inflammatory cycles produce extra transudate that leaks into tissues and isn't picked up and removed because the cycle is stuck. There is no transition to the next step and no true cleanup, which is the whole point of having an inflammatory response. The overabundance of neutrophils also wrecks that wonderful extracellular matrix (ECM) upon which new healthy tissue is supposed to be built.

A disordered inflammatory response, which happens more slowly but just as harmfully, is also responsible for much of the destruction associated with cancer. Though we often think of cancer as causing a wasting away of the body, known as cachexia, it is chronic inflammation that is the real culprit, not the actual cancer cells. The chronic inflammation of cancer causes every symptom we commonly see with its advancing stages—fatigue, pain, weight loss, loss of appetite, and weakness. The body is trying, and failing, to fight the cancer with an ongoing inflammatory response. The same thing happens with autoimmune diseases as the body literally turns its defenses on itself. It is well-meaning but deadly.

A second type of inflammatory overreaction during this first phase of healing is called disseminated intravascular coagulation (DIC). It is another central mechanism in severe COVID-19 illnesses and is often seen in times of critical traumatic injuries. Like a cytokine storm, it is a catastrophic event. It is triggered when the body senses either great blood loss or overwhelming infection. Basically, the body panics in its first wound response phase and kicks into high gear with all the defensive hemostasis-inflammatory response it can muster. In simple terms, it means that activation of clot formation and its fibrin mesh occurs inside blood vessels all through the body and all at the same time. It's as if the body's initial defense system received 911 calls from every location on the map. The problem is, when this all-out defensive response occurs everywhere at once, the body uses up all its platelets, and transudate leaks into all tissues. This causes blood pressure to fall precipitously. It is ominous and often fatal.

At one time, before medical professionals understood the roles of inflammatory blood components and how they called to one another, patients with DIC were treated with emergency fluids to respond to the leaks and blood pressure drops. As we've come to understand the interactions between inflammation and hemostasis in all aspects of early defense, DIC is better prevented and treated. Now patients are given equal parts blood, platelets, and plasma to replace those that the body produces and uses up. This may stop the body's overly defensive response so that the body can end its panic mode and continue to heal.

CR

The word *inflammation* comes from the Latin *inflammare*, which means "to set on fire with passion."[4] Our hearts are inflamed with passion when we fall in love; our words spark a roaring response when we provoke; our whole being erupts in a fit of rage when we react to perceived threats. For science to adopt this same language in the use of both acute inflammatory responses and the more maladaptive chronic ones is both fitting and curious.

It's not that our body burns us up when its inflammatory responses are properly controlled, but we do respond with redness, heat, and swelling. These cardinal signs resemble a hidden internal fire. Perhaps that gave rise to the term *inflammation* before we understood the molecular nature of it. Chronic inflammation, though less likely to display those cardinal signs, is more rightly a kind of setting the body on fire. Cachexia burns muscle tissue, consuming all that is good, relentlessly wasting and devouring us. Ulcers are like fire pits filled with smoldering embers, full of the debris of burned fuel and the ashes of old flesh.

Chronic inflammation is slow and insidious, not as externally dramatic as that Latin phrase implies. Despite its measured approach, once its fire has been fanned, it is almost unquenchable due to a steady supply of reinforcements from inflammatory cells. Like a small brush fire that starts in the dry Santa Ana winds of California, chronic inflammation rapidly explodes into a devouring monster. Whether a cytokine storm, DIC, or chronic ulcers, inflammation gone awry is very difficult to treat once it starts. We still have a long way to go in medicine to properly prevent these disorders from taking root.

And we still have a long way to go in our gathered lives as well. The disordered inflammation of our relational defense systems can destroy families, business partnerships, faith communities, and civil discourse. Those who experience the chronic stress of interpersonal conflict actually show higher rates of the biological markers of chronic inflammation, such as elevated levels of cortisol, adrenaline, cytokines, and dopamine. Here there is not just an analogy but a parallel relationship—those with communal chronic inflammation are at higher risk for heart disease, stroke, cancer, and early death than those without such stress markers.

Disordered inflammation has taken root so deeply in our social order that there is now a name for it. We are living in an *outrage culture*, which social scientists say is marked by an increasing emphasis on protest, division, and ongoing instability. Facebook posts ask us to sign petition after petition, demonstrators on bridges ask us to honk in protest of a leader, and our favorite fast-food place becomes a test of our allegiance to human justice. Memes of *OK Boomer* circulate as a ridicule of the older generation by the young. Outrage is so woven into the fabric of our society that it is becoming a knee-jerk response to anything done by a member of an opposing political party or someone of a different gender, social class, or ethnicity. Within the corporate body, the inflammation of chronic outrage releases more and more killer "enzymes" in a futile attempt to destroy a perceived enemy. As a result, the next stage of healing, discourse and the building of a platform together, is not even possible.

Whether expressed as a fierce storm or as a chronic response, protracted outrage also weakens the real need for selective outrage at the moral evils that threaten our neighbors' welfare. Habitual social outrage, in the sense of taking up cause after cause, may also mask one's own individual identity and unmet need for validation. Outrage's *heat*, says psychologist and author Dr. Terri Apter, speaks of "the dangerous pleasures of outrage,"[5] which cause us to feel morally superior. Because we feel so intensely, we reason we must be right and very different from those we protest! We like this expansive feeling and trigger it more and more, the dopamine response giving us a biological feedback loop, and we become increasingly intoxicated with confidence in our own superiority.

This kind of cultural outrage takes root insidiously, like chronic inflammation. Our initial response to an awful wound is often correct—a rapid strong defense is needed. When a rapid gathering can form a clot and limit bleeding, protest makes sense. But an inflammatory response becomes counterproductive when it becomes disordered and stuck in a repetitive, destructive cycle that doesn't address our wounds or allow the building of new life together.

Years ago, I was encouraged as I listened to a radio interview with a member of Congress. He was asked about his reaction to the large number of people around the country protesting a law that restricted some immigrant freedoms. He himself had voted against the legislation, thinking it unjust. The protesters were confronting lawmakers who supported the legislation, challenging them in restaurants, in front of their homes, and while they were with their family members.

His response surprised me. He asserted that people are entitled to peaceful protest and that he was grateful they were active in civic life. He said the protesters recognized that the immigrants affected by the law were their neighbors and deserved treatment as human beings worthy of dignity and respect. But, he added, the people with whom we disagree are also our neighbors and deserve the very same dignity and respect. He shared that taking this position—recognizing the dignity of those with whom he disagrees—stigmatizes him from some in his party, who think he should be more militantly separate from members of Congress with whom he differs. But his stance of controlled inflammation, limited to the topic and not generalized to a group of people, shows that he recognizes the warning signs of chronic inflammation and doesn't allow himself to become numbed by it.

If outrage is literally rage turned outward, another sort of disordered inflammation comes from redness, swelling, and heat turned inward. Habitual arguing, anger, and bitterness can settle deeply into our individual lives. Do we recognize the analogous neuropathies, hypoxias, ulcers, and cytokine releases that are present in our chronically inflamed relationships? If so, are there early warning signs for these, too, so we may prevent these disordered pathways from taking root?

Some time ago, I read a story about refugees who fled from a country where they were ethnic minorities. They had been persecuted for generations and denied land rights and education. They were victims of genocide and widespread brutal assaults. After a series of attacks, a strong eloquent religious leader of the minority arose, and the people cheered on his mostly peaceful protests.

When the demonstrations failed and the majority rule ramped up their persecution, the refugees fled with their charismatic leader in command. Amazingly, they arrived in the bordering country without significant loss of life. A safe zone of camps was established. At first, the people rejoiced as they hoped for lasting freedom from oppression. But then came news that their permanent resettlement would be delayed; they would continue to be confined to temporary camps far longer than expected. Their shelters were crowded and inadequate. Their daily rations were monotonous and far different from the food they were used to. The refugees started to argue among themselves about their best course of action.

Many complained that their old way of life was better than this one. At least back then they knew the enemy. They had left their familiar homes and traditions. Who could trust that the country where they would resettle would be any better? What if the new place was filled with people just as hostile as those they left behind? A small minority of refugees, faithful to the appointed leader, kept encouraging peace as panic and chaos increasingly swept the tent city.

You may recognize this as the story of the Israelites, led by Moses out of Egypt. They'd been slaves there, and through miracles of deliverance, they experienced an extraordinary rescue through the Red Sea on a journey to the Promised Land, said to be flowing with milk and honey. But it was a land route, not a direct flight, and traveling was difficult. The early wonders were replaced with some relative hardships—not slavery and persecution, mind you, just boring but sufficient food and a sweltering desert, yet with available water. Like a small splinter in the foot, this limited amount of discomfort started the chronic inflammation that would be the downfall of an entire generation.

This story is a powerful archetype for families and communities in relationship under stress. I remember the first time I read the story as an adult. I was stunned that the people complained so quickly after having just experienced so many jaw-dropping miracles. And this wasn't even their first time grumbling as a group—they had done it before in Egypt when they were unhappy with Moses.

Sadly, it seems most groups are quicker to complain than to encourage one another. In fact, grumbling and arguing is socially contagious. Like our body's defense system, once we initiate that first flare, it calls out for reinforcements. A cycle starts. And unless it rapidly ends with a clear transition to the next phase, the pattern continues to spread.

For some reason, positivity is harder to spread than negativity. It takes several positive statements to dampen the impact of one negative remark, according to the emerging science of positivity.[6] In the Israelites' case, Caleb and Joshua, two of those sent ahead to survey the Promised Land, saw it as wonderful, but the ten naysayers held sway over the minds of the people. The people of Israel had difficulty trusting in a better future, and the same is true in much of the world today. A Pew Research study found that the majority of Americans' distrust in government and in their interpersonal relationships has made resolving problems more difficult. Trust across ethnic groups, generations, and socioeconomic status differed considerably, with minorities, younger people, and those in poverty more distrustful than those in other categories. Fortunately, most respondents felt that the nation could improve trust by building avenues for collaborative public engagement.[7]

Lack of gratitude also seems to play a significant role in our biblical story, and it certainly shows up in today's cultural commentaries. This lack of appreciation focuses on what is missing rather than what is present and leads to a numbness, a neuropathy, to the complete truth. Lacking healthy perfusions of gratitude, our memory becomes impaired. Remember, remember, remember, say the biblical prophets.[8] It is a good reminder for us all.

BROKEN BONDS

Beyond numbing the memory and inflaming the mind with complaints, negativity leads to chronic arguing, which is marked by three characteristics. Those who argue incessantly assume they are never wrong, insist on things being just as they want them (generally impossible when it comes to other people), and place blame entirely on others.[9] The irony is that those three attitudes cause people to end up being more and more at odds with others, and so more rejected, exacerbating the chronicity. An insistent, unyielding posture results in self-sabotage, consuming healthy relationships as it spreads further and further, and isolating people more and more. Cachexia, amputations, and septic relationships are often the sad result.

Of all isolations, family separations are the most intensely personal. Family estrangement, in which there is unresolved conflict and no contact between certain family members, is measured at about 8 percent of the population in a large British study.[10] Another report reveals that about 10 percent of mother-child relationships in the United States experience this deep divide.[11] Further research in this area shows that over 40 percent of families have experienced at least some degree of family estrangement, often repeated through generations.[12] Although most of these separations resolve, the frequency of them within families is similar to the rates of divorce.

Research shows that family estrangements come from a

long, eroding, continual process. They are most commonly initiated by young adults ages twenty-four to thirty-five against their parents. Generally, these fractured relationships don't stem from abuse but from mismatched expectations and feelings of enduring pain and humiliation. Although it may come as a sudden surprise to parents when young adults no longer make contact, multiple factors lead to what psychologist Terri Apter calls "ruminating anger"[13] and the eventual split. Rumination, of course, is the physical process of redigesting food through fermentation, furthering breakdown. It is similar to the work of cytokines. Apter says the breaks in families cause "phantom limbs" and "never a scar, but always an open wound."[14] Both sides in the split are sad and confused.

The stark parallels between biological disordered inflammation and familial ongoing inflammation are tragic. Ruminating anger also calls to mind cachexia, the wasting away of muscle tissue. Consider the words of Frederick Buechner:

> Of the Seven Deadly Sins, anger is possibly the most fun. To lick your wounds, to smack your lips over grievances long past, to roll over your tongue the prospect of bitter confrontations still to come, to savor to the last toothsome morsel both the pain you are given and the pain you are giving back—in many ways it is a feast fit for a king. The chief drawback is that what you are wolfing down is yourself. The skeleton at the feast is you.[15]

As one who has experienced both sides of family estrangement, I know the anguish, stigma, and abiding sense of loss it engenders. My childhood was marked by my uncertainty of a parent's love for me, ultimately leading me to be as separate as possible during my early adult years. I missed holidays, birthdays, and other celebrations because of the trauma that overwhelmed me. I felt constant underlying grief. My siblings didn't necessarily have the same experiences or reactions, which is so often true. We couldn't really share our emotions about it even though we still maintained relationships outside of my parents' home. I was so ashamed of the situation, of the idea that as a young woman I couldn't bear to be near my parent, even though others in my family carried on normally. As a result, I hid the situation from as many people as possible. I often made excuses for the absence of a parent at significant events to avoid exposing the rupture.

Many people who experience this degree of alienation from a parent are wary of marriage and children. If they do have children, they often have only one. I wondered and worried about that myself, but my husband's love prevailed. We have five children, all of whom we love dearly. Yet it has not been completely rosy. In what I will always mark as one of the most devastating times of my motherhood, I also felt the grief of being on the other side of estrangement. One of my children felt the need, for her own sake, to break away from contact. At first I fought so hard against that. How? Why? No, no, no! It was unbearable. But after a while, I chose to just let her have her own life journey. I had communicated what I could. So I prayed for her health and peace daily. I prayed for her to know how deeply she was loved by God. I figured if that happened, the rest would take care of itself. And it has, for now. I've learned how tenuous deep relationships can be after a critical rupture. We still need to treat the wound tenderly, as it stays raw and painful when touched too firmly.

There is no simple process to prevent this devastating wound, and there are no quick remedies for its relief. The lesions of estrangement are complex and require our best efforts at long-term solutions, much as chronic ulcers do. I don't pretend to have the answer that everyone else has overlooked. But as we place our distress in the context of disordered inflammation, we are given some new imagery that may be helpful.

For a long time, cultural stigma prevented me from identifying this disease—ruptured relationships—in my life. No public posters described the sort of conflict I experienced. Even now, I don't see posted warning signs stating that chronic arguing and incessant demands can lead to an early death, yet the statistics are clear.[16] A friend who is a professional mediator and member of a faith community told me how rarely he observes people in small groups, even where they are known and supposedly safe, share the real struggles they experience in personal relationships. For example, lots of folks ask for prayer for a friend in the hospital but fewer ask for healing of a fractured family bond. The shame of our private battles keeps us from early interventions that could be lifesaving.

My Salem College alumnae group recently hosted a virtual spirit week. The ravage of COVID-19 had sapped our strength, and our alma mater, a small liberal arts college for women, was trying to buoy us up. At first, its Facebook page was flooded with happy pictures of students celebrating field days, dorm life, and other festivities. There was lots of silliness, and the posts kept coming. Then one alum commented that she ached when she saw these posts. She said she felt she had missed so much. While others were having fun, she remembers struggling during college with who she was, with her sense of worth and identity. She had been rejected at home and had questioned so much of herself. She yearned for a time capsule to take her back so she could participate in all the fun she saw in the photos.

Her comments instigated a second surge of activity. Many women admitted the same feelings. The popular girls, the scholars, and the leaders had deep struggles in college. The wealthy women who seemed so put together in their new clothes and fancy cars were often grieving a hidden sorrow. Family separations and self-doubt were everywhere, but they were kept isolated and private to avoid stigma. A collective sort of healing, a communal blessing, happened through those posts, which demonstrated that, in the end, we were more similar than different. It was the best college reunion I could imagine, a spirit week filled with the Spirit.

PUTTING OUT THE FIRE

In public health, we look for early warning signs of complications in a chronic disease like diabetes. We measure body mass index (BMI), a range of ideal weight for height, and we examine blood lipids, blood pressure, and changes in blood glucose. An HgbA1c is a marker of three months of the body's circulating glucose, and tracking it reveals how well-controlled diabetes is over time. People with diabetes also get annual eye exams and tests of their sensation in their feet. These are all indicators of overall diabetes control and whether patients are at risk for complications from chronic inflammation, such as the development of ulcers.

What are the analogous things we can monitor to avoid lapsing into habitual anger and outrage, whether it is caused by cultural forces or family estrangement? Who do we need to ask for help, despite the perceived stigma of admitting our problem? Just as an ideal BMI is a range that takes a while to reach for those who are obese or overweight, so curtailing ongoing inflammation will require adopting a range of exercises.

Every day we hear of new therapies on the horizon that will treat cancers and other difficult diseases with immunotherapy. This use of our natural immune processes seems like a wonder drug. What if we drew on some of our own "immune" resources (outlined below) to challenge the epidemic of disordered inflammation in our collective lives?

Practice positivity

There is no blood test to measure circulating levels of negativity. But there are a number of ways to track our moods and outlook, from smartphone apps to ancient spiritual practices. Mood tracking has been shown to help people manage anxiety and depression, and smartphone apps like Happyfeed and Moodistory make it pretty simple for the technology minded. Each day, people record their mood at a designated time. Then they reflect on their current state—they practice mindfulness. Looking back over a month, they can see what triggered certain feelings and then try to deal with them constructively. These apps really just do what old-fashioned journaling does.

I don't use an app, but I do practice an ancient low-tech discipline started by St. Ignatius of Loyola. Called the Examen, it consists of two questions to be asked daily (the Jesuits, started by St. Ignatius, practice it twice each day). The first question is: What are your consolations today? A consolation is a time when we think we drew closer to God, to our sense of rightness with the world, and to our sense of authentic self. Less formally, it is a spot of goodness, delight, or joy in the day.

The second question is: What are your desolations today? A desolation pulled us away from the ideal. It is a "not again" incident, a negative emotion or turmoil or outright sin. For me, it is a lost temper, a procrastination, or a refusal to yield to another's need. Sometimes it is working in a job that drains me, being part of a project that I don't feel suited for, or seeing that one activity is pulling me away from something better.

As we begin the Examen, we are to quietly become aware of God's presence with us. Then we review the day with gratitude. We attend to our emotions as we ponder how the day unfolded while contemplating our responses to the two questions.

The treasure of the Examen isn't held in a single day's recording. We are to review it over time and look for trends. What sorts of things brought consolations? How can I point my life more fully toward those? What things consistently show up in my desolations? How can I reduce those? Many people use this practice to discern vocations and other major life choices. In my case, it helped me see that writing was a gift to be given time, even if some might think it foolish at my age. It also helped me see that my chronic anger in certain areas of the medical workplace was due to the limits placed on practicing the kind of medicine I cherished, the kind that honors relationships and values each family in all of their humanity. Transitioning to different work environments has been joyful and life-giving as I accepted these desolations as markers of a deeper truth. These adjustments require risk as we must trust that something better awaits, even if it requires a costly change.

Another tradition is intercessory prayer. In the Sermon on the Mount, Jesus told the crowd, "Love your enemies and pray for those who persecute you" (Matthew 5:44).

Praying for those who persecute us is wiser advice than I first realized—it opens the way for restorative healing and limits chronic inflammation that results from negative rumination. It forces us to let go of the outrage, if only for a bit. And acknowledging our own neediness and struggles allows fresh perfusions of grace to reach our weak, weary tissues.

At first, I limited this prayer to only my fiercest critics. Once I saw how quickly it helped me quell my temper, I began trying to do it whenever I felt a sense of resentment rising up against someone. Anger at my neighbor's ineffective social distancing during the pandemic, despite repeated attempts on my part to control her, finally resulted in a prayer for her protection. She wasn't actually persecuting me. I was perhaps persecuting her. But engaging in this sort of prayer makes it almost impossible for me to stay annoyed.

Positivity literally expands our peripheral vision,[17] making us safer in places of conflict, like war zones, but also able to metaphorically see better, perhaps noticing the unspoken need of the person with whom we disagree. In another parallel to our analogy, positivity assists healing rates from surgeries and serious diseases. It is an essential component of a healthy defense system.[18]

Give in to gratitude

Count your blessings is not just a saying on a retro kitchen towel. Acknowledging what is good and beautiful leads to an internal perception of wellness, an attitude of joy, and an openness to others and their needs.

I keep a running list of things I'm grateful for, often looking at it when the current moment seems difficult or unjust. I have options for recording these little moments everywhere I look—a basket with a pen and slips of empty paper sits on a table in my office; a gratitude bowl given to me by a friend is in the living room, inviting others to write their reflections too; my journal is filled with consolations and desolations. A sign in my kitchen reminds our family of one of my early parenting refrains: "Attitude of Gratitude." During the pandemic, many people posted photos of beautiful landscapes or shared one grateful thought each day. There's no best method or secret to being grateful—practice makes perfect, and we all need practice.

Manage expectations

Most experts say that entrenched conflict is never solved by proving the correctness of an argument but is instead achieved by restoring a relationship. How much does "being right" matter versus moving toward a compromise, or reaching an adjusted outcome that promotes wound closure rather than amputation?

In terms of managing expectations, I love what my friend Julie always said when she invited folks to dinner. Because she had a large family of young children, guests invariably asked what they could bring to help with the meal. "Low expectations," Julie would reply, putting everyone at ease. Remember how the neutrophils expect their attack to destroy the wound problem, but they only make things worse when they continue fighting after they're no longer needed? In our chronic conflicts, we often deploy a similar weapon—wrong, rigid expectations. When we set those aside to identify what can actually be changed in the situation, we take a positive step toward healing. Sometimes all we have control over is our own assumptions. My expectations for myself are just as often a problem as the external issues are. One of my daughters painted a sign for me that now hangs in my office: "There is no way to be a perfect mom, but a million ways to be a good one." Amen! Lowering expectations doesn't mean lowering standards; it simply means allowing one another grace to heal and grow in the present reality of our circumstances.

Listen well

How much feeling is left in our chronically inflamed relationships? Like those skin patches in Hansen's disease, the neuropathy of rage numbs us to anything that isn't bent on destruction. Has our anger drowned out the quiet sounds of despair? Stopping to listen for the hurt of others takes great strength when the ulcers caused by constant agitation have already set in.

Listening is so countercultural that a new wave of writing and teaching on it has emerged as if it were a recent discovery. Listening is called an act of generosity, of love. It isn't a debate tactic; it is a recognition of shared humanity.[19] Rather than only presenting our own view in support of our arguments, we take the time to hear why a particular subject matters so deeply to the people we are with.

My family, like many others, finds that some of our most tense conflicts come from the mundane experiences of daily life. As a household that is now full of adults who come and go on their own schedules, we don't always take time to connect well when little things bother us. Personally, I get aggravated when I see clothes, books, and dishes left out. If I comment on this while everyone is rushing around, I quickly get hostile reactions.

Recently, we decided to sit down with each other and really try to work on solving these daily difficulties. We set ground rules, agreeing to listen to each other by allowing a five-second pause between speakers. We also allowed no interrupting. Even so, hands shot up, asking to be recognized next, while someone was still speaking. The next comment was already being formed in the listener's mind. This exercise wasn't easy for our verbal tribe! Yet we all agreed it was one of the best family meetings we have held because we refrained from giving our own opinions until we really listened to another's.

Counter stigma

The stigma of diseases like leprosy has been reduced through scientific and medical understanding, which has diminished the public's fear and given medical professionals clear guidelines on how to care for the afflicted. Many people who battle mental illness still think that seeking psychiatric help is a sign that their faith or willpower is weak; sometimes they fear that getting help of any kind means one is "crazy." None of us can overcome stigma singlehandedly, but the more we allow others to safely enter into our painful places, the less power that stigma may yield. The tricky part is knowing whom to trust. Some of us have bravely shared our struggles only to be rejected or misunderstood.

A mental health counselor named Gretchen Grappone writes about stigma from the point of view of her own struggle with depression and her work as a clinician. Overcoming stigma, says Grappone, starts with our own story and connects it with at least one other person's story.[20]

This is what happened in my college's Facebook posts. One person shared and others connected her story to theirs. Before we may feel safe to do this with those we know, anonymous sources may help. The National Alliance on Mental Illness (NAMI) has developed the documentary resource *In Our Own Voice* that openly examines the stigma experienced by a number of people with mental illnesses and includes examples of how those effects were overcome. Twelve-step support groups are beautiful examples of community alliances that crush stigma with unconditional support and friendship. Churches and other community organizations might follow suit by providing safe places for people to discuss some of their deep hurts, offering them solidarity as they are transparent about the struggles that all of us share.

My college is considering sharing our alumnae story with incoming freshmen to help them see that so much of what we may think is peculiar to us is actually a shared condition.

Of course, sharing without any follow-up can be worse than doing nothing. Protection of vulnerable hurting people is critical. The college will let students know about the resources available when they feel hurt, confused, or lonely.

Through the stories it tells, the media can also help alleviate the stigma we hold on to. Families have their own internal cultures. Mine didn't share deep hurts well, even though we handed them out like Halloween candy. Likewise, in a recent television episode of *This Is Us*, a kindly old doctor counseled Rebecca, a young mother who had lost one of her triplets at birth the year before. She felt shame for privately grieving her newborn when she had three living children. The doctor responded by telling his own story of loss—linking their life journeys. Physicians were once told not to do that; instead, we were advised to keep our distance. But he broke a stigma. His words were so moving; I tried to write them all down, and they go something like this:

> Hospitals [and life and families] . . . hold some of
> the greatest joys and the most awful tragedies all
> under one roof. I think the trick is not trying to keep
> the joys and the tragedies apart. Let them cozy up
> to each other. Let them coexist. And I think, if you
> can do that, if you can manage to forge ahead with
> all that joy and heartache mixed up together inside
> of you, never knowing which one's gonna get the
> upper hand, life has a way of shaking out to be more
> beautiful than tragic.[21]

When we've been badly hurt, our natural tendency is to avoid the people and situations that caused pain. If we perceive a new threat from the same source, our response may be rapid and explosive, a tempest. Our immune system, which is all about memory, behaves this way too. It stores molecular and cellular memories of past infections, as well as encounters with hostile intruders such as a foreign blood type or protein. When it experiences those a second time, it is ready with a much stronger inflammatory response. This is basically why tiny doses of vaccine can arm us against a real infection by the full disease.

When our immune system misreads the enemy, it may react against members of our own body with an autoimmune disease. In a similar way, we can use our past hurts to react against the possibility of health in our corporate body. Slowing our rapid defensive response in places of disordered inflammation allows us to determine if our reactions will promote destruction or healing in an ongoing wound. What good will our response produce? Is it drawing others in, supporting them, and weaving a healthy platform upon which relationships can be restored? Or will it just lead to more debris, more pressure, and a bigger collapsing mess?

Rapid correction of a wound is still important and the best defense. Ignoring an injury may lead to dysfunction. But when we habitually remember the good, acknowledge that everyone around us is fully human, listen well to those with opposing viewpoints, maintain reasonable expectations, avoid blame or the need to be right, and allow our wound to be open to healing, then the threat of a corporate wound becoming chronic lessens dramatically. By holding back the signal to release enzymes that will eat away at us, we get to work quickly so that new tissue that reaches across the two sides of a wound can begin to develop.

CHAPTER 4

VITAL CONNECTIONS

Collaboration and Community

Community doesn't just create abundance—community is
abundance. If we could learn that equation from the world
of nature, the human world might be transformed.
PARKER PALMER, *Let Your Life Speak*

ONE SULTRY SUMMER DAY while serving as medical director
of a migrant health center, I heard a pounding on our clinic
door. Two farmworkers were outside, holding up a third
man between them. That man was conscious but unsteady,
wearing long work pants, no shirt, no shoes, and no socks.
"Snakebite! Snakebite!" his friends yelled in Spanish. We
rushed the injured man into our treatment room.

Our clinic sat between acres of green, leafy tobacco and
rotating crops of cotton and sweet potatoes. From April
through November, over forty thousand farmworkers and
their families came to plant and harvest the fields, laboring
from sunrise to sunset six days a week in the North Carolina
heat and humidity.

I have never encountered laborers with a stronger work ethic. The workers lived by an unspoken code, something that was part of their culture and also part of their concern for survival: Never complain, and don't go to the doctor except as a last resort. Missing work meant missing pay. They reasoned that most ailments would eventually resolve on their own, or with help from a friend or a *curandero*, a traditional healer. A snakebite, though, could be deadly, and all the workers feared that.

The three workers had been sitting in a field, taking their lunch break. The victim told us that, as he sat on the ground shirtless and ate a sandwich, a copperhead had slithered up beside him, lunged forward, and bitten him on the belly. It was extremely important for us to know what type of snake bit him because in North Carolina some snakes are venomous and others are not. Antivenin was available, but it was also dangerous because its foreign proteins could cause a severe reaction. It would be available only in a hospital and was a very expensive treatment. We asked the worker if he were sure it was a copperhead. He insisted it was. As his wound was examined and cleaned, we explained about antivenin and asked again how he could be so sure it was a copperhead. He replied he knew because he had bitten the snake back.

The field-worker reached into his pants pocket and drew out the head of a snake. After the snake bit him, he seized it, bit it full force himself, and proceeded to kill it with his bare hands. It *was* a copperhead. An eye for an eye, and a bite for a bite.

The snake had bitten him in the best of all possible places on the human body. The abdomen has loads of room for swelling. (Every pregnant woman knows that.) Though the venom did seep into his tissues, it didn't go far. His abdomen blew up like a balloon, but we gave him lots of IV fluid, managed his pain, and he did well without needing antivenin or an expensive hospital stay.

The worst part about snakebites is that most happen on hands, feet, arms, and legs. These locations have what are known as compartments. The muscles and tendons are encased in neatly separated sheaths wrapped by thin strong fibrous tissue called fascia, which is like a strong plastic wrap. The fascia keeps everything wrapped snugly in a bundle, which helps each muscle grouping move as a unit and makes mechanical sense. The problem is, there just isn't any extra room in those compartments, and the venom and swelling often become trapped, intensifying the injury. The initial inflammatory response has nowhere to go with the transudate, unable to moderate the growing pressure it is creating in such a tight space. As the transudate pressure increasingly pushes down on the healthy muscles and nerves, it rises in force until it crushes them. This disastrous effect is called compartment syndrome.

When a venomous snakebite happens in an arm or leg, no matter how well the person looks initially, they need to be moved to an emergency facility as quickly as possible. If swelling starts in a compartmented area, time to treatment is critically important. Emergency teams actually repeatedly measure the tissue pressure inside the swollen region with needles hooked to pressure gauges. If the pressure gets too high, it will kill surrounding tissue, causing irreversible neuromuscular damage. The pain is exquisite as the area's blood supply gets cut off, the oxygen delivery to the tissues falls, and the pressure builds. This entire event can happen in four to six hours, which for a farmworker in a rural field can be the blink of an eye.

Penetrating injuries caused by machinery are another type of occupational injury seen on farms. In these wounds, motor oil is another terrible menace to the tissues. Whenever compartment syndrome occurs, venom, particles in the wound space, or infections can create serious complications.

A crude but limb-saving technique to avoid permanent destruction by compartment syndrome is to flay open the fascial sheath containing the muscle, nerve, cartilage, and tendons, thereby relieving the pressure. In extreme emergency cases, such as battlefield sites or remote locations, the procedure can even be done outside the hospital. Sensation in the limb is largely lost by that point, and creating a long open wound immediately relieves the pressure, allowing drainage to start and healing to begin.

Most often, this procedure—called a fasciotomy—is performed in a sterile operating room. The compartments are cut open with a long incision, irrigated, and thoroughly cleaned of any debris that may cause further damage. The injured area is then left split apart without closing the incision. Though the body's hemostasis and inflammation crew have already been at work, the inflammatory response needs assistance from the surgical team and antibiotics.

After a fasciotomy, surgeons delay closing the wound so compartment syndrome won't reoccur and the injured area has time to recover from the pressure of inflammation. The wound is tended with dressings and sometimes with a wound vac, a little vacuum that sucks out debris and keeps the site clean. Several days may go by before a decision is made as to how to close the wound. Sometimes the body allows the closure to occur as healing progresses, with rapidly decreased swelling. But if the wound is large, a skin graft may be needed. Occasionally, traction devices are used to stretch the skin, expanding it to cover the gap made in surgery. The goal is for new tissue to fill in the wound site as much as possible, and for function of the limb to be preserved.

No matter the procedure chosen, the fact that people heal after fasciotomy with function, tissue growth, and healthy skin covering their wound is incredible. It is not only a tribute to well-coordinated teams of medical professionals, but also to countless molecules and cells signaling, responding, joining, and dying as they collaborate in a matrix of cooperation more elegant and sophisticated than any we orchestrate as hospital specialists.

This phase of wound healing is called tissue regeneration and repair. Its chief of staff is the extracellular matrix (ECM). The ECM is material like biological superglue or a giant sticky spider web. It is secreted outside the cells and acts to hold the cells together in a certain formation, like a scaffold or a 3D building framework. In addition, the ECM serves as a communication superhighway for processes in and out of the cells.

Unlike a human chief of staff, the ECM, which we shall also refer to as the healing matrix, isn't really a singular or even a static unit. It is a scaffold upon which to build but also a dynamic, constantly changing collection of molecules supporting the surrounding cells. If a scaffold, it is one made for flexibility in construction, as it adapts its shape to whatever is best for the body in the environment in which it finds itself. It continues to alter throughout one's life, from fetus to old age, and throughout life's experiences, from health into sickness or injury and back into health again. Within each organ or tissue, the healing matrix differentiates to best meet local needs. Not only does it adapt to its locale, but the cells with which the healing matrix interacts also act upon it and change it in that process.

Scientists like Bem know there is enough complexity to the healing matrix that one could study it for a lifetime, but we will get to know it here more simply as it responds to a fasciotomy. Suppose a farmworker is bitten on the calf. Within hours of the bite, the pressure of the wound will almost destroy the healing matrix, as the body tries unsuccessfully to direct the inflammatory response to stop the crushing swelling. At this point, the patient will need to undergo a fasciotomy. During the procedure, the release of pressure and cleansing saline irrigations are like a refreshing shower, helping the healing matrix reassemble and get back to work. Three days after surgery, out of sight of the medical team, the healing matrix is busily working inside the wound.

There is so much cross talk going on between the tissue cells and the matrix molecules at the fasciotomy site, it's a wonder the surgeons can't hear them. The cells in the wounded tissue have receptors for the healing matrix on them, like little ports that can plug into the matrix hard drive and get a message. There is also a wireless feature, as signals are sent by the healing matrix through enzymes to helper cells elsewhere in the body to come and join the building process. All of this communication directs cells to migrate into new places for new work, to replace injured and dead cells, to multiply and build new blood vessels, and in all these ways, to rapidly support new tissue growth.

Fibroblasts, cells that start the growth of new fibrous tissues, are in the wound site. They have gotten the message to secrete fibronectin, a sticky protein building block. Like a spiderweb, the healing matrix scaffold is being constructed out of this fibronectin, which had been largely inactive before the signals came for its production. Fibronectin gets most of its use in the embryo stage of life, when there is a rapid need for building new tissue. Later, it is used in forming that sticky gauze in clots, as well as in matrix web construction during wound healing.

Fibronectin is a supportive team member. It literally lies down like a net and allows other members of the body's healing team to crawl all over it, assisting cell migration, adhesion, and growth. It helps the binding of collagen molecules, fibrin (its stronger counterpart), and integrin. Integrin is a real hotshot, something we will come back to in a moment. The binding of these molecules makes a platform for new granulation tissue, the initial tissue to form in recovering wounds. Granulation tissue is full of tiny nourishing blood vessels. A plump soft pink pad, it is like a living gauze bandage at the wound site.

The healing matrix releases cytokines, but these aren't destructive like those overproduced in chronic inflammation. These are used as a wireless communication feature. They signal for help to cells all over the body, which come and participate in the tissue-building process. Pretty soon, all sorts of cells are migrating to the matrix, where it is rapidly becoming crowded. It's a good thing that the fasciotomy opened up a lot of space. Before long, the surgeons will see evidence of what is going on in there.

The integrin that binds to fibronectin in the matrix is considered a hotshot because it has a job similar to what you might see at airports. Like those workers who use a little cart to pull a huge empty plane into a parking space on the tarmac, integrin guides the lineup of new tissues. It sticks to the matrix platform, like a cart on the tarmac, but it also latches on to the incoming tissue cells, guiding these newly forming cells to make up the walls of capillaries and muscle fibers. It gets them to position themselves properly so they form tubes for blood vessels and fibers for muscle. It helps them bend and change shape and arrange themselves in three dimensions to assure we don't end up with newly clogged capillaries or fibers that are patterned like a cornfield maze. It's a good thing medical science doesn't have to figure out this level of repair!

Meanwhile, with all the crowding and shifting of cells into new positions, there is some tension in the healing matrix. But in this instance, some tension is good. It signals to the wound that tissue is growing and the soft pink underbelly needs some mature muscle to be formed. This tension also signals that those cells that have completed their defense work need to die. Programmed cell death, called apoptosis, is triggered by this wound stress and makes room for appropriate scar or tissue growth rather than a mound of difficult immature tissue that inhibits function.

Apoptosis, along with the tension of the pulling tissue as it remodels and grows tighter, is a process that takes time. In the case of a fasciotomy, this reshaping is often helped by surgery, but the body still has to do most of the work behind the scenes. Remodeling at the molecular level happens over months and even years until the shape conforms to the function it is to serve. In this phase of wound healing, plans both for engaging community collaboration and for ceasing such efforts have to be in place at the same time, with constant attention to the balance of both processes. In a supportive environment specially constructed for each individual wound setting, all sorts of cell types must do their parts at just the right times, in response to chemical, electrical, and mechanical signals.

Finally, the snakebite wound suffered by our fasciotomy

friend has healed. Though scarred, his limb moves as it should and his muscles are strengthening. His feeling is intact. He is able to live a full life despite the visible reminder of past pain. He brags to everyone about his amazing medical team at the hospital. The healing matrix sends out sarcastic signals about going on strike next time.

ℭℜ

One year, two of my young adult children faced serious illnesses at the same time. Hospitalizations were frequent and unpredictable. My work included travel twice a month to review the performance of public health clinics throughout the country. Despite always being on alert for an incoming call from a family member, I was fully engaged with my colleagues at the clinics as I reviewed their sites. Coworkers who knew of the times where I needed to step out to take a call or rearrange travel to go to a hospital commented on my focus at work. I told them I could compartmentalize. Work was actually a relief as it gave me an opportunity to fully concentrate on what was before me and not to ruminate on scary possibilities that might overtake my children. That sort of compartmentalization in our corporate life is considered a healthy defense mechanism. We have our own fascia bundles surrounding the various ways we need to show up, and usually they stay nicely in their own separate spaces.

Psychologists discuss another sort of compartmentalization, which gets mixed reviews. I've experienced that, too. As a child, when a frightening adult repeatedly overpowered me, I detached emotionally. I compartmentalized as much as possible so that at a subconscious level, I did not allow my whole self to become injured. Instead of hearing what was said in a way that allowed it to be recalled, words were heard but not recorded in my memory. My ears were full of a rushing sound as I felt myself close up to the outburst before me. My efforts at compartmentalizing weren't a total success, and I carried trauma into the future. As an adult, when I was in the presence of that person, I still detached, going to a different space I couldn't articulate. It was an odd experience, almost feeling as if I were watching myself in a movie. I wanted to respond but felt numb. I didn't understand it until it was explained to me. I was too good at compartmentalizing, whisking away my entire presence in the room when faced with that stress.

These types of compartmentalization, which require counseling from psychologists and other therapists to help address, are just as much part of our individual makeup as our muscle bundles are. However, there is another kind of compartment syndrome that is often not recognized until late in the process. It can be deadly as it overtakes and crushes our corporate wounds. I've seen this in sudden traumas, such as when a loved one dies in a car wreck and the fault lies with the driver, who is sometimes a relative or close friend. Shock sets in, then anger. Sometimes there is a clamoring from many sides on the proper course of action, the best next steps to take. Meanwhile, the loss is profound and not able to be grieved well. The venom from the conflict has gone into a space that can't breathe, where there is so much pressure from a strong inflammatory response that the pain is unbearable. Those who are supposed to be helping are only making matters worse with their inciting responses and urgent questions. We need our collective healing matrix to be opened and freed, so that healing, rather than amputation or death of relationships, can occur.

On the world stage, we see this type of compartment syndrome all the time, as bundles of people experience the crushing effects of sociopolitical wounds without a community matrix in place to promote healing, or even regeneration. Closer to home, partisan politics can also act like one of the body's compartmentalized tissue sheaths. If operating healthily, all groups, despite their separate areas of emphasis, pull toward a goal that benefits the whole body. But too often, we see multiple separate compartments, weakened by venom and unable to draw on the diverse community of the body for life-giving support. In our faith communities and families, our pressure gauges may show we need intervention, but it isn't always clear that there is an underlying matrix of support poised to respond.

CLEARING THE CLUTTER

Most of us have people we can quickly call upon when we've been deeply wounded. They are our first line of defense, serving as our "clots" and providing a healthy inflammatory response. Some may stop our initial hurt and stabilize us.

Others may acknowledge the crisis at hand and respond with righteous indignation. They offer whatever support they can muster. But if that support fails to clear out debris left by the wound, we may feel increasing amounts of anger, resentment, and frustration. Our defensiveness becomes deadly when it crushes our ability to respond to others in a patient, adaptable way. If all we have in these painful situations is a group of like-minded defenders who tightly gather around us, we may never be reshaped into healthy, functioning members of a body larger than ourselves.

So what tools can we draw upon to promote the regeneration of community?

Practice mediation

Sometimes we have to flay open the wound. It is usually our last desperate effort after other methods have failed. Both the injured ones and the community healers must agree to the process. The suffering have to be able to trust that those holding the knife are competent, skilled in healing, wise, and committed to their well-being. Many times, painful past experiences prevent such trust. Just as our farmworkers generally avoided physicians, so the seriously wounded in our communities may avoid our ready outreach.

Mediation is a practice marked by such a flaying. It brings together two sides that haven't been able to reconcile and who often don't trust one another's intentions. Sometimes, there is a clear victim and a definite perpetrator. Other times, there is just ongoing animosity around an unresolved issue. A professional mediator told me the story of an older woman who had been robbed. The thieves were young teens responding to a dare. The boys were caught and faced charges for theft. Routine courtroom litigation could have quickly resulted in justice, with the adolescents locked up and the woman made aware that they were punished for her distress. But real healing required more.

Mediation was needed. Each side had to come together not only to tell their story, but also to listen. The woman told the teens that, although she was not hurt during the crime, her fear of another attack was crippling. She had become unable to leave her house. The victim wanted to know why they had targeted her, why she was preyed upon. She desired assurance that they would not do it again. Mediators say this is a common question among injured parties. The simple answer from the teens was just that she was caught up in a crime of convenience. She was not recognized as a person with fears, but as an object with a purse. The boys were not trying to terrorize; they were trying to get approval from their peers. As a result, they faced criminal records for impulsive acts, which would damage their future options. They explained that they never meant to cause permanent damage.

As the woman and the teens saw the human beings behind the crime, they could let go of the deadening behaviors that were destroying their ability to flourish. Justice could take place as restoration rather than retribution. The teens were still punished, but they were also truly contrite for causing harm they had never imagined. And the victim felt heard, consoled, and restored.

Mediation practices such as these are decreasing the rates of reoffenders in juvenile justice. Recidivism is about 20 percent for youth undergoing mediation, as opposed to about 40 percent for those in traditional courts.[1] My mediator friend Don Lotz points out that vulnerability, diversity, trust, growth, and sacrifice give way in mediation to lasting healing. Volunteers as well as paid mediators may act as a bridge between the parties, establishing a safe neutral space where there is clarity identifying what happened and why. Mediators are like the fibronectin net, laying down a scaffold upon which new tissue can be built.

Don explains that behind the scenes, the tactics are complex, involving a number of critical steps. The process looks simple on the surface, but much effort goes into readying the victim, managing time and emotion, avoiding revictimization, and allowing the full story to unfold. The mediator first meets with the injured party and then separately with the ones who caused harm. The fears and perspectives of all parties are given voice. Then their concerns about the process are answered. Rules are made clear: There should be no screaming, the meetings will be in a safe space, and the elephant in the room—the real wound—is named. The truth is not hidden. Through this process, both sides develop trust in the mediator.

Like the situation in a healing matrix, the local environment changes with the case at hand. Mediators need to adapt to the circumstances in each individual setting in order to promote the best outcome. Sometimes people need only one session, sometimes several. Sometimes family members are present, other times it is very private. When the process works well, mediators testify that the healing is palpable. They watch as faces soften, shoulders drop, heads come up, voices change timbre, and eye contact is made. Don notes, "All speak of what they know, fear, acknowledge, regret, and hope for." Rather than viewing justice as an incision to remove an unwanted lesion, it becomes instead a space suited for new growth and for inclusion back into community.

Mediation is used formally by the courts for both criminal and civil complaints. Many people use it in the process of divorce proceedings and child custody. But it also is widely used in workplace conflicts. Professional mediators may be lawyers, therapists, or others trained specifically in mediation. A number of associations exist, including some that are specifically geared to faith-based situations. Jewish, Christian, and Islamic mediation organizations all draw on similar scriptural principles and use similar techniques.

Embrace diversity

When the one hundredth anniversary of Nelson Mandela's birth was observed in 2018, many wrote of his accomplishments, which included helping end apartheid in South Africa and becoming that nation's first black president in 1994. Some people also reflected on how his efforts were grounded in his own particular experiences. His life was informed both by his father's Bantu tribal teachings and his mother's Christian faith and education. His prison guards included white members of groups oppressed by more dominant Anglo colonizers, which encouraged Mandela to reflect upon injustice as a universal human experience rather than merely factional. A favorite saying of Mandela's was from the Bantu culture: "We are people through other people." He insisted that the African National Congress, the political party he led, be multicultural and multireligious with mutual interdependence. "The common ground," he said, "is greater and more enduring than the differences that divide."[2] For Mandela, generations of wounds in South Africa required a healing matrix marked by adaptation, diversity, tension, and even an apoptosis—the destruction of racial segregation.

One way that Mandela's legacy lives on is in the Prison-to-College Pipeline program. Initiated in New York by Dr. Baz Dreisinger, it recognizes the crucial link between education and safe communities.[3] The program offers prisoners access to higher education, mentorship, and community support to prepare them for employment after their release. Rather than a one-way prisoner-to-society reform effort, the Prison-to-College Pipeline recognizes that prisoners have something to contribute to other university students as they interact within the campus setting. The program is active in New York, Mississippi, the United Kingdom, Jamaica, Trinidad, and now in a South African prison similar to one where Mandela served time.

A 2013 report noted that those who participate in education while incarcerated are 43 percent less likely to return to prison than those who don't.[4] The underlying hope is that reforms in criminal justice like these will include a narrative shift about prisons and those who are incarcerated. Like the integrin latching on to cell after cell in order to shape a blood vessel correctly, classes and guidance from mentors for inmates build and support a new shape for life outside the prison.

In ways similar to Mandela's, author and speaker Parker Palmer calls us to heal the heart of democracy. His reflections are strikingly analogous to the function of the healing matrix. Palmer writes, "When *all* of our talk about politics is either technical or strategic, to say nothing of partisan and polarizing, we loosen or sever the human connections on which empathy, accountability, and democracy itself depend."[5] He names five interlocking habits necessary for healing our wounded efforts at democracy:

- We must understand that we are all in this together.
- We must develop an appreciation of the value of "otherness."
- We must cultivate the ability to hold tension in life-giving ways.
- We must generate a sense of personal voice and agency.
- We must strengthen our capacity to create community.[6]

Like the healing matrix, these habits rely on establishing a local platform upon which to give and receive assistance from diverse groups, allowing tension to be a signal for further growth. Individuality is preserved even as community shapes the whole. As we began navigating the COVID-19 pandemic, we gained a fresh understanding of our interdependence upon each other. The old and fragile relied on the young and strong to avoid contagion. The health workers depended upon the sanitation workers, and everyone depended upon the farm laborers. All were called to sacrifice something for the good of another, and tension did build as we were stretched into new ways of interacting with one another. Many preexisting arrangements for meeting the individual needs of people, whether for food, medicine, comfort, worship opportunities, or even companionship in death, had to be built anew.

Our essential workers acted as fibronectin, laying themselves down so that others could be healed or kept safe. Early on, nurses and respiratory therapists traveled from distant places to serve spots in crisis, acting as those mediator cells that come from afar. When the crisis was calmed, the mediators dispersed. The push and pull of allowing public life to continue while also protecting the safety of the community took on vital importance as we tried to understand the appropriate tension needed for healing. And new communities grew—virtually, locally, and across what previously might have been some factious lines. "Stronger together" is not just a catchphrase of a pandemic: It is a truth in building up a healed humanity.

While new life appears in wound healing, death is there

as well, as we leave behind the ideas, attitudes, and actions that are no longer of benefit in our reshaped lives. Many of us realized what we could live without as we lived through the era of COVID-19. All of us, whether wealthy or poor, conservative or liberal, young or old, shared our vulnerability. When a healing matrix takes a firm hold, human connections are ultimately preserved and strengthened while less important matters are swept away.

Palmer contends that it takes not just intellect, but also emotion, self-image, and a shared sense of meaning for these habits to flourish.[7] This reminds us of the greater instruction to gather together our whole selves in the love of God and neighbor. In the Jewish tradition, the *Shema* is the great call to acknowledge and love the Lord with all of one's being.

In Judaism, the *Shema* mystically unites fellow Jews with each other and with G_d as it is recited. The 248 words in the Hebrew recitation are said to correspond to the 248 "limbs" in the male body, loosely associated with bones; in ancient times, rabbis imagined the body with 248 limbs and 365 tendons. Linking the number of words with the number of limbs, Jewish teaching says that the completion of the prayer brings healing to the whole body. But in order to get to 248 words, the *Shema* includes the ending where all join in and say, "The Breath of Life is our Source" (*Adonai Eloheichem Emet*). For that reason, fullness in the recitation of the *Shema* is possible only when the individual voice is joined in with the wider community as they praise the Holy One.[8]

Christians are similarly taught that there are two great and corresponding commands: to love the Lord with all of our heart, soul, mind, and strength; and to love our neighbors as ourselves.[9] The individual habits that shape our being give way to a corporate shape of humanity as we join in imaging God. During the start of the pandemic, Christians worldwide prayed the Lord's Prayer at noon their time each day. Praying in unison in this way served as a large fibrin mesh that all of us could join. As these prayers are lived, they provide healing to our individual spirit as well as to our mystical body of Christ. The healing matrix imagery, in a practical sense, shows us the many ways love is an actualization rather than an abstraction so that wounds are not allowed to fester. Love takes place locally in many different environments and situations, with neighbors we don't always recognize or wish for. It is characterized by unity in diversity, every member contributing according to the gifts they have been given, laying themselves down for the sake of others, and ultimately giving way to death for new life to take shape.

Invite others in

Modeling the idea of working to fully close all areas of a wound, Sister Simone Campbell, a Roman Catholic nun, lawyer, and activist, practices contemplative listening as a way to promote complete healing. Sometimes called "soul inquiry," contemplative listening is an effort to pay attention not just to what is said, but to what is meant. What is the truth behind the words? For Christians, it seeks to recognize the presence of the Holy Spirit in the conversation being shared. It is patient and nonanxious in approach, allowing the speaker to unfold their story as they are able, without criticism.

Sister Simone resists the idea that we can only be concerned about the 99 percent when the one percent seem culpable for an injury. Whether that one percent are the billionaires, the sports stars, or the most murderous of inmates, she prays to understand them so that all of us can be folded together into a seamless healthy body. Wounds left gaping, even if only by one percent, will never fully heal.[10]

What might this look like in our social healing? How about those enzymes that call out from the healing matrix for cells, those far removed from the injured site, to join the process? They may have played no part in creating the injury or allowing it to fester. Yet they belong to the solution; indeed, they are necessary to it.

As I have worked in many cross-cultural settings, it has been delightful to learn about the manners and traditions of others. Cultural differences, if not recognized, have an enormous impact on the effectiveness of public health and medical interventions. In recent years, this has become better understood and incorporated into the education of most health professionals.

As a writer and teacher, I've taught many sessions on cultural competence, better termed cultural humility. We sometimes employ an imaginal technique called the Table of Significant Others (TOSO). Participants are asked to close their eyes and imagine they are seated at a dinner table, surrounded by those people who are significant in shaping their decisions and views. Whom would they want at their table if facing a crisis? If trying to resolve a deep struggle? Or to shape their future endeavors? At this point, they can pick anyone they find significant in their life.

For most of us, the TOSO exercise reveals that our tables are full of people who are generally like ourselves. Socioeconomic status, race, ethnicity, politics, gender, religion, profession, education, and age all tend to separate us from others. It is no simple task to remake our tables so that those foreign to us become known as dinner companions. But when that occurs, we are apt to find that we learn exponentially more about ways we may interact to promote health and well-being. How can we invite some new enzymes into our wounded places? Of course, it is best if they are already present in our healthy spots.

People don't instantly come to your table if asked. Recall that trust is most impaired in those who are members of a minority group, in poverty, or of a younger age. If someone is asked to a table so that a quota is filled, they will sense that. So first, those who hold a seat at the table must ask themselves if they are attacking the real problem. Then they must decide if they are still best for the table. After these questions are answered, invitations can go for others to join in.

I've seen some great examples of this play out in community health centers that serve the marginalized. Most of the clinics are directed by a board of directors, with some of the positions automatically reserved for experts in finance, government, and health care. But the boards also have positions for experts in the lives the marginalized patients lead—the homeless, the HIV infected, the migrant laborer, and others. These patients are representative of the mission of the center, and without their active engagement, the center can quickly be blind to barriers that keep people from accessing care.

For instance, homeless board members have helped clinic administrators understand that patients need to be in line for evening shelter by late afternoon, so they can't keep appointments that are scheduled then. Immigrant members helped a center realize that when doctors dressed casually, rather than making the patients comfortable, it made them wary of the doctor's skill. Immigrant use of the emergency department had increased because the doctors in the hospital all wore white coats. It really didn't have to do with hours of access or cost or other things that were initially thought to be the issue.

One center in Maine asked their community to identify unmet needs and barriers to care. They asked patients what they would like to see developed at the center. Then they established small groups, called Circles of Concern, that were open to those interested in the topic. As underlying problems dealing with stigma, patient perception, and cost of care were unearthed, so too were groups of people willing to work constructively on the issues. Creativity and enthusiasm flourished.

In my own life, my patients and colleagues have been great teachers. As a young doctor, I explained to a teenage mother how she could use time-out as a disciplinary practice. She asked me how *she* could do this. She lived in one room with a number of farmworkers. She didn't want her child to upset the others or to be out of her reach. I realized how little I knew. On consultant travel with colleagues, I watch as they worry about the rental car and the license tags. I see them avoid even the slightest traffic violation. I sit in the back at night as police pull over my Black friend for not using his turn signal at a stop sign on a deserted road. I learn how being a minority affects so much of daily life.

Regeneration and repair cannot be compartmentalized. We must allow an open space for others, inviting them to set up shop on the foundations of our very selves so that we may be refashioned. We are made, down to our fibronectin biochemistry, for community. We are never really one, as individuals. Mysteriously, we echo that concept of the Trinity, one yet three, separate yet in a reciprocal dance that cannot be divided or destroyed. Signals we don't fully comprehend call us to one another, linking us together and applying a process of tension, release, and death to our wounded places as we patiently participate in a new shape that fits the form and function of shalom.

CHAPTER 5

PROUD FLESH

Necessary Rewounding

"Knowledge" puffs up, but love builds up.

1 CORINTHIANS 8:1

ONE OF MY FAVORITE PATIENTS on the island of Molokai was Lani. At two years of age, she was a testament to the love of her teenage mother and the resiliency of newborn life. Her entry into this world was catastrophic; because she did not receive enough oxygen during birth, she suffered a stroke, which led to extended time in intensive care, numerous surgeries, and repeated near-death episodes. All her organ systems were damaged, and no one could predict her future development or life span. Her care included multiple medications that had to be monitored weekly, a feeding tube into her stomach that provided all her nutrition, and daily therapies to keep her muscles limber. Despite all the strikes against her, she flourished in surprising ways, always coming into the clinic with a broad smile, ready to show off a newly acquired skill. She genuinely enjoyed her interactions with our staff as we cared for her and caressed her, and she responded with delight to the affection of her mother.

In the midst of Lani's major medical obstacles, her mother had the most difficulty with one thing that seemed trivial upon casual observation. The tissue around the baby's gastrostomy tube—the tube going into her stomach for feeding—was pink, thick, and weepy. Sometimes the tube leaked a little, and the nearby tissue bled whenever it was rubbed. Though it stayed bandaged and clean, it was always puffy and wet. It just refused to heal into a dry scar. The soppy bandages chafed Lani's skin and stained her clothes with yellowish spots.

That problem at the tube's surgical wound site is called excess granulation tissue. It is a fairly common complication that happens when a wound is constantly irritated by friction or doesn't get enough nutrients and oxygen. The healing is stuck in the early stage of tissue repair, and so this new connective tissue just keeps growing, continuing even beyond the boundaries of the wound edges. The excess granulation tissue somehow switches off the migration of epithelial cells, which are the components of skin. Typically, the movement of epithelial cells is like the closing of elevator doors over the wound opening; both sides move steadily toward the middle until the gap is sealed. Without that migration, the covering layer of skin can't be formed.

Instead, a useless lump of flesh is formed that extends outside the original wound edges.

A slang term for this overgrowth of granulation tissue is *proud flesh*. This term reflects its British origins, where to be proud can mean to project up and out from the rest of the group or to be so swollen as to stand out from the rest. The phrase *stuck up* has a similar meaning. Such projection and swelling is always interpreted as foolish rather than dignified. In wounds, proud flesh is weak and unhealthy, made mostly of capillaries, white blood cells, and fibroblasts. It bleeds and is easily infected, is always wet, and lacks the protective surface epithelial cells would provide. It delays wound healing and causes chronic problems that often require surgeries to remove the extra granulation tissue. Though this may sound more like an ugly nuisance than a serious threat, proud flesh can be deadly. It affects all mammals and is one of the more common serious complications known to affect the legs of horses, often resulting in a lethal wound. Because this overabundance of granular tissue spreads past the wound's boundary, it prevents proper closure of the wound.

Wounds that result in proud flesh get the first part of healing right, but once granulation tissue begins to form, that phase of healing doesn't stop. The healing matrix is then unable to help pull the ends together in closure. The community portion of building and signaling that gives tensile strength to scars as they form is lost.

We tried to deaden Lani's extra tissue using silver nitrate applications on a regular basis. Silver nitrate sticks look like matchsticks, and when they touch the wet tissue, they form a reaction that cauterizes, or burns away, unhealthy tissue. Because there are no nerves in granulation tissue, it doesn't hurt. Unfortunately, that treatment didn't work for Lani. We gave it time, and then we sent her back to the surgeon. He cut away the excess tissue and forced the wound site to start the healing process all over again. Sometimes repaired wounds still form proud flesh, but in Lani's case, she healed. That problem, at least, was solved.

CR

When comparing physical and corporate healing, "proud flesh" hits particularly close to home. A wound is present and raw, but it has stopped bleeding. The initial inflammation has quieted down. We start to lay a foundation upon which to build resolution. However, this is where the trouble begins. In the case of interpersonal wounds, instead of drawing on the help of others, we attempt to patch up the hurting space using only our own limited resources.

Like Lani's small gastrostomy tube site, those bits of proud flesh may look insignificant at first glance, especially when compared to everything else we are dealing with and what we have already overcome. But even those minor granulations are threatening irritants that can infect the way we think and feel, leading to further injury and requiring determined removal if we ever want wholeness and closure.

Yet as much as we may want a relationship mended, we

may find it difficult to relinquish full control of the situation, even when that is needed for further resolution. As a result, our original complaint stretches into what had been healthy areas. We may make a mess of those areas while obstructing healing of the original problem.

We've all been taught that in a fair fight, we should stick to the boundaries of our current argument. We are not meant to bring up past problems or expand the issue with generalizations that paint everything with a negative brush:

"You are always the one who is angry about issues."
"That is such a white male perspective!"
"What about the time you didn't respond to my request for help with the finances?"
"Even if you are sorry now, you didn't seem sorry when you misled everyone last year."

Sweeping accusations like these are frequently the cause of chronic unhealed wounds. Sometimes we even lose sight of the original problem because all we can see now is the lump of proud flesh expanding past the wound site.

Family fights over inheritances can lead to accusations about favoritism, love, and manipulation rather than recognition that a parent chose to dole out material goods in a way that may be painful for some recipients. Soon the siblings view each other—rather than the deceased parent—as the traitors. In churches, different understandings about who is qualified to serve in leadership can cause not just wounds, but massive amounts of useless proud flesh, when the two sides make hateful accusations attacking the integrity, faith, and Christian love of the other.

How often do we find ourselves, after the initial crisis of a wounding has passed, vowing to make sure we will never allow ourselves to be in a position for that to happen again? We build up our defenses, thinking we are making ourselves strong against those we still perceive as foes. It's quite a challenge to stick to our proper boundary lines, but it is the only way for healthy repair. The two sides of a wound need to meet with a clean edge, and that requires a bridge to be built. In physical wounds, this connection is created by a community of cells that come into the wound and work on new tissue formation. In our corporate lives, this happens by allowing the imposition of others in our community to help resolve the rupture. Keeping our boundaries clean isn't a one-time thing. It requires constant discipline to avoid our granulation making, trusting we won't be destroyed by what is meant to help us heal. The irony is, if we don't limit our defensive postures, we may very well be destroyed.

Often, differences in our social settings create an unspoken friction when unplanned events demand our attention. Resentments arise at work when employees with children leave promptly for day-care pickup while those without children stay late. The irritation may increase when holiday leave is approved more often for those with children at home or those who need to travel. When allowances are made once, everyone is generally happy to help. But when exceptions recur, employees may feel growing ill will toward coworkers with children, so much so that hiring decisions may be affected. "Remember when all those people left at five o'clock the day before the grant was due? Let's not get into that situation again."

When hiring, organizations can then be skewed toward the preferences of those without family responsibilities. Instead of working on how to handle the ebb and flow of unanticipated problems with a diverse group of employees, the issue is avoided. I recall experiencing this when a male practice partner advised I talk "skirt to skirt" with female pediatricians about how to handle family responsibilities while taking a call. His tactic didn't prevent the overflow issues of family compositions, day-care needs, and conflict within an intergenerational workplace from forming granulation tissue in our office. Meanwhile, wounds between those with family needs and those without grew deeper, with both sides feeling pain.

Similarly, single people often feel left out when decisions are based upon the majority who are coupled. Faith communities often experience this tension, and it is no wonder that there are so many separate styles of worship services and small groups based on similarities rather than differences, despite calls for unity within congregations.

I experienced tension as a mother who worked part-time, never fitting in with the stay-at-home group that dominated my church. I felt hurt at being automatically excluded from groups they formed. Couldn't they at least ask me to join and let me respond? In my defensiveness, I felt proud that I spent more hours a day with my children than they did, since they went to clubs and volunteered and socialized while baby-sitters or preschools watched their children. *And anyway,* I told myself, *those groups are a waste of time.* In proud flesh, we think that a good offense is our best defense.

Unfortunately, in medicine and in life, we usually don't know that proud flesh is forming until we are well along in our granulation process. Our relationship may appear healthy at the beginning. We seem to be on the right path until something sets off an overreaction.

LIMITING FRICTION

In the science of wounds, we know that the lack of sufficient oxygen, the presence of chronic disease, and anything that causes friction to a wound—rubs it the wrong way—may interfere with proper granulation and lead to proud flesh. In our corporate wounded places that are still raw and just beginning to heal, we need to watch for anxiety, despair, anger, and depression. These classically rob us of openness to the ideas of others and insight into our situation; it is this receptivity that may act as our breaths of fresh air and oxygen.

Our chronic cumulative losses and hurts may surface again with each new wound. They have to be guarded against so that they don't shape the new situation abnormally. And it is all too easy to be rubbed the wrong way, allowing another unhealthy layer to form that will need to be trimmed so that reconciliation can take place. There are several steps we can take to prevent proud flesh from taking hold.

Catch and release

This saying applies not only to fishing; it is a good phrase for keeping proud flesh at bay. If we find that we are forming just a bit of proud flesh, we must act decisively to destroy it. The key is early detection of that unhealthy impulse to spread beyond our designated borders, so it can be stopped and redirected with a minimum of disruption. While in the world of biology there are no nerves in the granulation tissue, in the world of our corporate hurts, we may feel like one giant twitching neuron. It will hurt to remove that proud flesh. For young Lani, we tried silver nitrate sticks in an attempt to burn away the tissue overgrowth. For us, it may take a daily discipline of meditation, prayer, confession, or contact with a trusted partner to help eradicate and prevent harmful overgrowth.

I have a friend who is starting a new missional community for those who have largely been outside of the church; some have even been rejected by those within it. He started this endeavor with vision and hope, certain that new, healthy tissue could be formed in wounded places. A discernment process acted like the initial granulation layer. Then as he was inviting others to help him take the next steps, he kept trying to articulate what his community would and would not look like. As he did so, he had a sudden realization.

Despite professing a generous love for the church, his references to other church gatherings repeatedly took on negative connotations. The joy and gladness of gathering with a group of people out of a sense of love and belief was overshadowed by growing criticism of established methods elsewhere. Proud flesh was forming, interrupting what had begun as a journey toward wholeness. Growth was reactionary rather than centered on building a fresh model of missional community.

My friend's response has become an iconic image for me in picturing the practice of cauterizing emerging proud flesh. Through accountability and spiritual disciplines, he became aware of how his tone and emphasis had shifted as he led the creation of this new community. Because he'd overstepped his boundaries, his focus had become disordered, and the community was losing the shape of the original tender tissue. As a corrective, he decided to abstain from negativity for thirty days. That abstinence, like the daily silver nitrate sticks, eroded the newly formed proud flesh. By the end of the month, his focus was renewed, his joy returned, and the work went forward.

Allow the scalpel if necessary

In the medical realm, proud flesh has to be removed, and the wound rewounded for appropriate healing to take place. Rewounding is typically necessary to destroy proud flesh when it has settled in, becoming a chronic irritant. When we see that we've spread beyond the boundaries of our corporate wounds by bringing in immaterial and unhelpful issues, we have to stop, acknowledge those matters and the damage they are doing, and remove them. It isn't something that can be done in secret by the offending party—the acknowledgment of our misstep must be public, as the revision of the wound will be. If it's hard to avoid forming proud flesh, it's harder still to deal with it once it has formed.

In this era of social media, some posts that aren't meant to be political end up as galvanizing when comments link them to one ideology or another. Several times, I have seen a friend of mine post what was meant as a helpful comment, only to receive a flurry of negative remarks about her beliefs and attitudes. She generally is gracious and ignores inflammatory language. While she is clear about her stance on social issues, she wants to stick to the subject at hand. What impresses me more than her silence in the face of ridicule is her willingness to accept correction, even from an apparent foe, when she is proven wrong. A public figure was roundly criticized for a supposed moral failure, and she shared that news online. But when some of her detractors pointed out that the story had been twisted, she quickly posted a retraction and an apology. This willingness to keep her boundary lines clean, and to be open to the voices of those with whom she disagrees, makes me pay close attention to what she writes. I trust her because of her integrity and her refusal to become reactionary in conflict.

What does rewounding look like in our corporate situations? It may involve therapy, mediation, assistance with past trauma, and an acknowledgment of our own role in preventing complete healing. In cases of great injustice, whole communities must come together to hear real apologies and accept reparations before any wound closure is possible. The Truth and Reconciliation Commission in South Africa, which heard from both victims and perpetrators of apartheid, is regarded as a successful example of such community rewounding in the name of ultimate healing.[1]

In our chronic wounds with family, community members, or workplace associates, it is challenging to allow the removal of proud flesh. I know that sometimes I have not been ready for the scalpel. I never did confront my friends about how hurtful their selective exclusion of me from their social groups felt. When we give up our claims, we can feel fearful, particularly because the outcome is often unclear. When time and energy are in short supply, we may prefer to keep things as they are. A weepy chronic wound is a known element. Before allowing the wound to be reopened, we want to believe that those who have wounded us will respond if we take drastic vulnerable measures toward real healing.

At this point, Jesus' question to a suffering man may be appropriate. The Gospel of John includes the story of the lame man who lay on a mat by a pool of water traditionally thought to have healing powers.[2] When the water was stirred—perhaps by a temple priest of the cult of Asclepius, Greek god of healing—people would rush to be the first one in. It was believed that healing occurred to those who entered just as the waters were stirred.

Jesus asked the lame man if he wanted to be healed.

Presumably a beggar, this man had been seeking healing at the pool for decades. He never seemed to make it to the water in time. The man responded that he did want healing, but he blamed the crowds and his inability to get to the water in time as the reasons for remaining disabled. There were too many obstacles for him to overcome on his own, so he still sat by the edge of the pool.

Jesus then simply told him to pick up his mat and walk. He didn't need the water, the temple, or anything else. Such a simple command must have seemed absurd after all the time he'd spent focusing on the obstacles to healing. But the man did as he was told, and he walked! Who knows, perhaps Jesus asked the same question of many of the wounded folks there and only this man took him up on it. The lame man risked being seen as a fool and had to be willing to give up an identity that was defined by hardship.

It may be simpler, at least in the short run, for us to interrupt the healing process and stay in the wounded place. Healing may require a lot of change—and a lot of humility to burn away our proud flesh. In a perverse way, we may enjoy our proud flesh, as it is an obvious reminder of how we've been wronged. How might our life change if we let go of everything that we uselessly carry around? I wonder how the lame man's life was changed when suddenly he no longer lay helplessly near the pool.

In removing our proud flesh, we may need to go back to square one. We have to choose repentance over pride, focus on the current issue over other wrongs, promote the community's welfare over self-righteousness, and acknowledge the other's boundaries over our own sense of wider margins. We must be shaped anew in ways we cannot fully control, ultimately joining forces with those on the other side of our wound more fully than we thought possible.

Keep the wound boundaries clean

Boundaries are odd things. Many are sites of contention rather than healing. We make boundaries to decide who is in and who is out. We separate and take sides. When we own property, our boundary lines tell us how much space we have between our neighbors, who are only welcome on our side of the line if we invite them. As parents, we tell our children not to cross that line! When a therapist says someone has poor boundaries, it is not a compliment. Human boundaries are about ownership, rights, and personal identity.

The natural inclination is to think of unpleasant restrictions when we think of boundaries. It is even like being *bound*. Rather than enjoying our boundary lines as places of refuge and safety, we often see our boundary lines as limiting—places of challenge, fear, and conflict. We operate from a sense of scarcity, wanting more. Wars are fought over boundary lines. Walls are built. Captives are taken.

But we can see boundaries either as hemming us in or as giving us freedom. In Psalm 16, David takes this second perspective. He says that the boundary lines have fallen for him in pleasant places and that he has a delightful inheritance.[3] Yet this is a psalm spoken in the context of danger. David recites this as he is being pursued by enemies who want to kill him! He is uncertain of his kingdom and his future in it. It's not as if he just won the lottery and he is saying a nice thank-you to God.

How and why does David say this? As a member of the tribe of Judah, David is heir to land that borders enemy territory and contains large tracts of wilderness. This strategic portion of land has been promised to the Jews through God's covenant with them, but constant attacks from neighboring ethnic groups seem to challenge the reality of that covenant promise. David is relying on his memory when every circumstance tells him he is doomed. He rises above the present conflict by recalling what has been promised to him and trusting in God's ongoing faithfulness. He knows where his boundary lines begin and end.

Like David, I try to trust my boundary lines when life seems to be spinning out of control. It is too easy to seek security or support beyond where I'm meant to be, especially in a hard and hurtful situation. In my own life, family and work have sometimes been places where I've questioned my boundary lines and inheritance. I've wanted some expansion to my limits—to belong to a certain group, to be noticed for my sacrifices, to live a certain lifestyle. I've also suffered losses that make me wonder about any sense of goodness ahead—deaths of family members, rejections at work, and betrayal in leadership positions. There have been some deep wounds along the way. They've been full of friction and left me gasping for air. Those are perfect conditions for proud flesh to develop.

In those times, I've learned that visualizing the limits of the wound is helpful. There is only so much damage that can happen in any situation unless we choose to perpetuate and expand it. Perhaps it is true in some sense that others can make things worse, but it isn't necessarily true in an emotional and spiritual sense. Nothing can remove the image of God from us, or the value of what it means to be ourselves, bound by our own unique expression of humanity.

When we stop reacting to perceived wounds that spill beyond our healthy boundary lines, we may see our injury with more clarity. We need to ask, What is the real problem that needs to be healed? Do we *want* it to be healed? What excuses are we giving for remaining immobilized as we contemplate problems that are beyond our ability to resolve?

God's understanding of boundaries and inheritance is very different from ours. Despite the fact that he is master, he doesn't give us the portion of a serf but of a noble person and family heir. He gives us his own portion, which is beyond description. He is bound by love, not by fear. He desires to unite rather than divide.

How are we to understand God's boundaries for us? We need a helpful image of God, and of ourselves in God. Voltaire is said to have noted that "God is a sphere whose center is everywhere and circumference nowhere." We are invited to dwell, to abide, in that center. We are called into the very center of what Christians understand as the Trinity, where all that is true and real is spread like a feast before us, and there is always enough, always more love to share, always more generosity for those in need. In that center there are no limits. No fears. No walls. No captives. There is only grace.

Richard Rohr writes on the mystery of the Trinity and the life of the Christian who finds herself centered in God. He says, "Traveling the road of healthy religion . . . will lead to calmly held boundaries, which need neither to be defended constantly nor abdicated in the name of 'friendship.' This road is a 'narrow road that few travel upon' (Matthew 7:14). It . . . emerges only when you hold the tension of opposites. Note that *holding* does not usually mean completely reconciling the differences."[4]

Those centered in Christ, Rohr says, "are paradoxically risk-takers and reformists [with] no private agendas to protect. Their security and identity are founded in God. [They] can move beyond self-interest and fear. . . . Because they have learned to live from their center in God, they know which boundaries are worth maintaining and which can be surrendered, although it is this very struggle that often constitutes their deepest 'dark nights.'"[5]

We are not supposed to think of ourselves more highly than we ought; yet we are also to value each other as beloved children of God. That is surely a paradox. Perhaps in loving our neighbor we will find the way to love ourselves. This is truly centering. Instead of a demanding knowledge or a useless pompous pride that puffs us up, we will discover a love that builds up, drawing healing to the margins that await our care and binding together what has been divided.

CHAPTER 6

SCARRING AND MATURATION

Form and Function

*Let perseverance finish its work so that you may be
mature and complete, not lacking anything.*

JAMES 1:4, NIV

PHYSICIANS ARE TAUGHT TO START with the chief complaint. As succinctly as possible, we ask patients to tell us why they have come to see us, and then we dutifully enter that information into their charts. Sometime later, toward the end of the visit, we record a diagnosis, our ultimate statement about what we think the visit revealed. The chief complaint and diagnosis are bookends to visits that often last only fifteen minutes. A cadre of staff designated as coders and billers read our records and make sure the chief complaint and the diagnosis are both entered so insurance companies will promptly pay their invoices. If either the complaint or diagnosis is missing, the chart is sent back to us so we can fill in that vital information.

In all my years of medicine, I've never seen an analysis showing how often the chief complaint actually matches the diagnosis. I suspect it is only a fifty-fifty proposition. Patients, though compliantly reciting their chief complaint, often wait until they are safe within an exam room to reveal their more worrisome symptoms. Sometimes their concerns have to be drawn out over several visits. As I have cared for people across cultures and age ranges, I have come to believe the term *chief complaint* is a misnomer—better to call it an opening volley.

Adolescents are particularly good at giving tidbits of information, separated by silences or shrugs, one morsel at a time, much like Gretel leaving a trail of bread crumbs to map her way back home. That was my experience with Josie when I met her in an urban clinic. A high school sophomore, she repeatedly came in with her father, usually complaining of a sore throat and earache. She never had a fever and always seemed healthy.

Only when her father left the room as I perfunctorily performed an annual physical could I see that she had not yet given us her actual chief complaint. I asked Josie about her goals, her school, and her daily life. Like many of the children at that clinic, she was being raised by a single parent. With tears in her eyes, she told me that her mother, who was addicted to drugs, had abandoned the family when she was eleven. She had a lot of questions for me—questions a girl would ask a woman, a mother, and a doctor.

When I had Josie pull up her shirt so I could better listen

to her heart, I noticed the scars. Just under the bra line and down her left armpit, I saw two-inch-long lines of puffy tissue, one after another after another. Some crisscrossed; some seemed to stack up together. She cast her eyes down as I looked at her. Next I lifted her limp arms, rolling up the sleeves of her baggy sweatshirt. The lines on her forearms were fresher, still with pink ridges and specks of dried blood. Hot tears fell down Josie's face.

Our time for her diagnosed "well child physical" was almost up. Josie gave me permission to call a therapist and get her into confidential counseling. At fifteen, she could see me as her pediatrician without parental consent if the problem concerned sexual or mental health. But she had worried her father would object, and so she had kept returning to the clinic without revealing the real source of her pain. As we worked together over the next few months, I told her she could call for an appointment to see me anytime, and she could provide my staff with any chief complaint she wanted. I would always see her, giving her space to let us know her real needs. Her father did eventually learn the full story and supported her need for therapy. Josie's angry, raw stripes slowly faded, and taut white tissue took their place.

I have become good at asking about and looking for self-harm. It is never a chief complaint. I don't recall hearing of cutting in my youth, but today's teens are quite aware of the practice. It affects both boys and girls, becoming prevalent even as early as middle school. So many times now, I've seen the visible reminders of a traumatic childhood—upper thighs with too many scars to count, abdomens with fresh wounds on top of raised pearly marks from bygone struggles—as my patients' faces look still and forlorn. My patients tell me they have to cut deeper and deeper to be soothed. We almost always embrace.

Scars are often the only visible signs of our past wounds, the default healing mechanism that signals our body's completion of its efforts to repair our injured spaces. Scarring and remodeling mark the final stage of wound healing, happening over months or years instead of the few seconds it takes to make the first clot formation.

With all the beauty and collaboration involved in the first three phases of healing, this last step seems a limited response and a gross disappointment to a process that so vigorously promotes restoration. But this is where the pragmatic and long-term responsibilities of the body's systems come into play as they seek to provide closure and preserve function. Regeneration is usually not possible beyond fetal development, so scarring offers a chance at protection from infection, restoration of strength, and further engagement with life without the body continuing to expend resources on past wounds. Scarring is a survival mechanism.

Let's reconsider those flesh wounds endured by Josie. Since they were mostly small and superficial, her body could quickly move through clotting, inflammation, and tissue proliferation. Very little angiogenesis (the formation of new blood vessels) was needed, and no muscle or nerve had been destroyed. Fibroblasts helped form granulation tissue and laid down type III collagen, a protein fiber that is packaged in multiple strong strands and made the wound site puffy and thick. Myofibroblasts, like elastic cords, helped contract the wound so that closure could more readily take place. Most of the cells used to clean up, fill in, and stabilize the wound then died and were removed by apoptosis, the term for programmed cell death.

Next the collagen was remodeled for a smooth closure to seal off the wound. This process reminds me of the way we used to construct a craft I loved at summer camp. We made lanyards out of long plastic strings, braiding them together into a design, three strands at a time. Eventually, we joined those braids into a rope. Likewise, in scar formation, collagen molecules, which are a braid of three strands of protein, join together to form a fibril; fibrils then join together to form a fiber. Strands are integrated into strands and into bigger strands. If a cord of three is not easily broken, as the proverb goes, then a cord of collagen fibers is pretty indestructible.

As the scar develops, the fibrin ropes transform into tighter strands by losing water—they go from type III collagen to type I, allowing the strands to pack together in compact layers and cross-link. These stronger type I cords align across tension lines in the skin, giving order and enabling the new scar to bend and twist in the same direction as the natural movements of the body. I never thought much about this until I was a medical student, trying to bandage wounds.

Bandages pop right off if they aren't aligned along the tension lines. Fortunately, our bodies don't make such rookie mistakes.

Scars lay down collagen in bundles parallel to the skin, increasing tensile strength, allowing the scar to be pulled tightly without breaking. This idea of maximizing tensile strength is another thing I'd hadn't considered before studying medicine—it's incredible how the body can make a tight new covering with just the right amount of force—not so weak that the scar is floppy and not so tight that it snaps in half. It's much like sewing a fine seam on a garment, making sure it creates closure but doesn't pucker and buckle.

In the end, about 80 percent of a scar is transformed into the tighter type I collagen, while the rest remains the puffier and softer type III collagen. Similarly, a scar will give the wounded area back about 80 percent of its strength. Scars don't contain the other parts of skin, like hair follicles and sweat glands.

In wound healing, the simple presence of a scar does not signify full success. The scar must be flexible, adaptable to the site, and stable over time. It has to be free of debris and allow normal function of the body. Remodeling is required as the scar ages.

Remodeling happens over a long period of time. By their nature, scars are slow to yield their original shapes. They were survival mechanisms, after all. They did well in getting us past that original wound, so any new effort at shaping is met with some resistance. In the physical body, such reshaping is triggered by the pull of healthy tissues on the scar. The scar is molded to adapt to the needs of the whole so that function is maximized. Even in physical wound healing, the seemingly visible repair is not the last word. Sometimes, surgical revisions must occur to aid the body's natural processes. Physical therapy is often necessary to help the scar become a supple component of the body, able to act in concert with the tissues surrounding it. For serious wounds, functional healing may take months or years. An ideal scar works well within its bodily location, doesn't create new problems with its presence, and generally allows life to go forward in an uninterrupted manner.

୦ଷ

In medicine, we pay attention to the wound environment, which is its relationship to the rest of the body, particularly those parts with which it will be in closest contact. Will the scar be over a joint that needs to move? Perhaps it will be across the upper back, where the normal tissue is pulled tight and smooth. Or will it be within the body, adjacent to organs such as the intestine and liver, where it may tug and bend as it heals? To support healthy scarring, we seek to relieve excess tension, avoid infection, and guide the ultimate shape of the scar. We have to patiently wait for the body to engage in remodeling. Sometimes, genetic disorders associated with scar formation make the healing process lengthier and more complex.

RESILIENCE AND REMODELING

If scarring is a healthy final response to most wounds, a way to provide closure and permit optimal continued function, how might we envision this phase of healing in our corporate life? How can we ensure that scars are flexible, adaptable, and stable? How do we allow for any remodeling that may be necessary in the future?

Uncover the true chief complaint

Even though a group may be unified in their desire for healing, it's possible that our collective diagnosis misses the underlying assumptions of the problem. One way to get clarity is to borrow a method I learned from a friend. She evaluates large grants and helps organizations shape their strategies to solve key problems. In framing the work, she asks a simple question: What will define success for you? Not only does the answer look to the future with hope, it is aimed at addressing the underlying problem.

During the COVID-19 pandemic, we saw communities struggle with how to move forward in ways that allowed full form and function. A deep wound had not yet been healed. Tension pulled on the puffy patches of recovery. Some people wanted to resume life as if the viral scourge never happened. Many were worried that their economic hardships would overwhelm them more than any infection might. Others drew back, eyeing the more carefree as potentially contagious threats.

It is important to hear the valid fears, concerns, and struggles that each member of the community faces, not just in the midst of the virus, but in the context of what will become a scar in our historical life together. Just as in the inflammatory stage, any leftover debris needs clearing—this is another opportunity for all voices to be clearly heard, a checkpoint before we move on at last. We have to be able to pull together in the same direction, somehow getting just the right mix of tension—enough to smooth over the wound, but not so much that it will snap. Recovery at this stage necessitates getting to an agreement on what success looks like, knowing that it will still take the shape of a scar, a permanent change from the pre-pandemic corporate life.

Allow scars to tell their stories

In relational and social conflicts, our scars must be acknowledged. We have to accept that most healing is accompanied by scarring. This is not a sign of failure, but a compromise made for the good of the whole. How are our corporate scars labeled? Are they trophies of a battle won? Humiliating signs of stigma and conflict? Or a map of memory, marking both deep hurt and profound recovery?

This step shouldn't be undertaken too soon. Wounds that are raw can hurt when touched and still be difficult for others to see. Some sidewalk wisdom suggests that we "share scars but not wounds." The idea is to share what we've learned or give counsel to others from the standpoint of looking back after gaining some experience and reprieve. Wounds need to be covered and kept from bleeding. Scars show resolution and healing. Sharing our raw wounds is a necessary way of getting support and care early on. Sharing scars is a way of testifying to the healing and the journey that unfolded along the way.[1]

Corporately understanding our scars may reduce the tension in the underlying wound, minimizing new scar formation and infected ways of thinking. Invitations to communal dialogue may give shape to smoother and more organized layers of repair, rather than a chaotic stranding together of disparate voices creating an ultimately weak patch on a complex social situation.

I've seen this struggle to give scar formation its rightful place in corporate healing portrayed in responses to war memorials. Protesters want to tear down those memorials that seem to glorify an abusive past. Other people counter that the memorials are appropriate since they convey how the past was understood, and we can't be revisionist. While recent controversies center around memorials to Confederates and former slave owners, the Vietnam Veterans Memorial is an example of the vitriolic response that deep wounding can generate.

Though it is widely admired now, the Vietnam memorial was highly controversial before, during, and immediately after construction. Inspired by a Vietnam veteran's distress over the scorn heaped on his fellow veterans when they returned to the States, the memorial would acknowledge the sacrifices these men and women had made and provide solace to those who made it home. A national competition for the architectural design was held, and the entries were reviewed anonymously, their creators' accolades unknown to the jury of architects and artists.

The planners required that the Vietnam memorial be apolitical in nature, but the war itself sparked some of America's most passionate—and at times violent—political protests. How could a memorial possibly speak to all affected by this fresh wound in American history?

The winning plan, selected from nearly 1,500 submissions, was drawn by Maya Lin, a Yale University student and daughter of Chinese immigrants. While walking on campus, she had been moved whenever she saw the names of alumni lost to war, which were etched on the walls of a rotunda. Her plan was in shocking contrast to other war memorials. Erected in 1982, the monument, constructed of somber black granite sunken deep into a green field, bears more than 58,000 names—all those who died or went missing in action during that war.[2]

At first, many protested the memorial's design, saying it was really a symbol of dissent and not of honor. But from the moment it opened to the public, the site became a sacred spot, a place of solemn remembrance and love for all who suffered. It did not celebrate, but it did remember and honor. In the end, this symbol of such deep division and pain was used to unite and heal.

Most of the ruptures we experience in our lives together are not on the magnitude of national strife. How might we see our communal scars as healthy remembrances of healing and perseverance, our own sort of memorial? The ancient Israelites provide an image that has been helpful in my own life—an Ebenezer. When Samuel and his army defeated the Philistines in battle, Samuel took a stone and set it up as a memorial, calling it an Ebenezer, or stone of help.[3] He did this so that when the Israelites saw it, they would remember that the Lord had helped them right to that point.

My battles are often due to my own faults, rather than to those of others. But when a struggling season ends and a healing time comes, I sometimes choose a stone from the beach and place it in a pottery bowl on my shelf as a remembrance. Later, when discouraged or worn out, I can look and see how far the Lord has helped me come, and continue on.

During a conflict within my church, the whole congregation wrestled through weighty issues of social, political, and theological conflict. We did the first phases of healing well—clotting, appropriate inflammation, and tissue building. When it was time for closure, the tension increased, just as it does with scar formation. Not everyone was ready to move on, but for the good of the body, we did. Recognizing the journey that had taken place, one that included loss of membership, grief, and conflict, this season in our church life closed with a service of lamentation.

All who had been affected by the conflict were asked to take part, including those who had left. We gathered together and named our collective experience. We each were given a piece of cloth, a symbol of our individual struggle. Then, each strip was collected and bound together, creating a whole fabric. That fabric was draped over the cross, remaining there for some time as a sign, a scar, of remembrance.

Get the tensile strength right

In the fairy tale of "Goldilocks and the Three Bears," Goldilocks tries out the bear family's chairs, porridge, and beds until she finds ones that are neither too big, too small, too hot, too cold, too hard, or too soft. She wants her experience to be just right. So, too, our corporate bodily scars need to be neither too soft, too tight, too thick, nor too fragile. In physical wounds, we rely on fibers braiding together, changing composition and adapting to the shape of the surrounding tissue. In our collective wounds, how might we mimic this transformation of tensile strength and fiber formation?

One possibility is to examine who is responsible for leading the closure. Is it an individual or a group? Does the leadership reflect the character of the injured? Sometimes in our rush to resolve a conflict, we announce that the past is the past and declare that we should focus on the future. These closures can feel sudden and instantaneous if there is still a freshness to the scarring. I've seen this premature completion of a complex situation more times than not, whether at work, home, church, or in the community. Patience runs out, even though we are so close to healthy resolution. Rather than all of us laying down our hurts and getting the tension to a healthy spot, we get a tightly bound scar, with no flexibility at all.

It is definitely important to get closure and move on from our conflicts. But in this last phase, understanding how to achieve healthy tension as scarring proceeds is critical. If the closure is too abrupt, the fibril bands of community are stretched too tautly. Under tension, they snap. People leave the corporate body, thinking healing just isn't possible despite all the formal efforts that preceded this last step. More damage ensues, with fresh wounds.

I saw this recently at a health center where I had worked. Money and time had been spent on responding to systemic problems in the workforce, but after getting everything out in the open, eliciting community participation, and making some positive changes, the leadership prematurely closed further attempts at reform. Multiple resignations ensued over the following year, with the company experiencing fresh repetitive wounds that required new resources to address. If we allow diversity in closure, with patient layering together of what we understand is bound up in our scar formation, we have a better chance of creating an Ebenezer for the community that will long be remembered.

Anticipate patient remodeling

In the human body, complete healing doesn't happen in isolation and never occurs with just one type of cell or protein. If it did, all our scars would be composed of disorganized strands that don't pull together. At best, they would be lumpy patches of mixed-up collagen. Scars need to have healthy tissue tugging on them in order to be rightly formed. So too, as conflicts heal and scars take shape during resolution, we must be open to continued work to keep that area of bodily life fit. When we feel our old injuries tugged upon in a new situation, it's a good time to reflect on whether that pull is meant for our harm or for our well-being.

Our social lexicon is full of words that deal with the scars of past trauma. Commonly heard is the term *trigger*. We are triggered by situations that remind us of past pain. They take us back to the original injury, trapping us in anxiety, anger, or depression. Generally, being triggered is considered a bad thing, and we try hard to prevent former suffering from having any voice in our present.

However, there can be beneficial triggers as well. They can be reminders that we still have some work to do in order to continue our healing success. For me, this sort of prompt often occurs in situations where I am with people who have been braided into my scarring places. They, or someone near them, make a comment that alerts me to a potentially charged situation. It's like a tingle in a nerve, or a yank on a resting muscle. If I allow that energy to pull me closer to them, I give my scar a chance to become even more adapted to a future that functions well in their midst.

For example, after a very long season of anguish with one of my children, we finally made it through all the stages of healing such that we could point to our scarred places with love and tenderness. I was—and still am to an extent— cautious about doing anything to disrupt that alignment of tensile strength covering past hurt. But gradually I am learning that when my child says something that strikes me as a potential point of conflict, it can be an opportunity to stretch a bit more into even greater unity. By asking clarifying questions, listening well, and letting my child know the parts in the discourse that are hard for me to understand, we deepen our respect for each other's differences even as we maintain our own individuality. Rather than being satisfied with a superficial but safe relationship, we probe areas of faith, politics, sexuality, and identity together in a manner I never would have thought possible.

Such remodeling is slow but beautiful as we integrate our scar into the healthy body of family, and ultimately, into our collective image of God. Just as our body heals at a micro level in order to promote wellness at the macro level, so attending to our personal scars as they integrate into our lives may assist us as we address society's collective scars as well.

CHAPTER 7

IMPAIRED SCARRING

Distortion and Contracture

*Have you ever been hurt, and the place tries to heal a bit,
and you just pull the scar off of it over and over again?*

ROSA PARKS

WHEN MY FRIEND SHANNON had an emergency Cesarean section, she stopped the obstetrician on the way to the operating room. "Promise me you'll be sure I end up with a discreet, barely noticeable scar." He laughed and told her she'd be left with a baby as the chief outcome, but the doctor did say he'd do his best. In truth, much of how we scar is out of the physician's hands. Shannon's request wasn't made out of distrust or vanity; instead, she had a collagen disorder that left her with scars more pronounced than most. Other people have genetic abnormalities leading to keloid scars or causing prolonged wound healing, problems that invite infection and complications that may interrupt scar formation.

Two types of scars are problematic, sometimes requiring medical help for their revision. Hypertrophic scars are larger and thicker than normal; some cause contractures, pulling too forcefully on adjoining tissues, which limits the range of motion. These are more likely to form when a wound becomes infected or the closure happens with too much tension, either due to the surgeon's procedure or because of the wound's location. For example, scars across the upper chest and shoulders require high tension to close a gap from a wound. Repeated signals from the body to increase tension can cause scar overgrowth and thickening. Hypertrophic scars form with too much type III collagen, making them puffier.

Keloid scars also cause trouble. They form due to an exaggerated healing response by the body, which causes the scar to balloon well beyond the borders of the wound. They are caused by errors in the body's own wound-healing mechanisms, preventing the disorganized collagen from being shaped into an orderly array of parallel mature fibers. Unlike normal scars, keloids form with lots of elastin, which makes them weaker. Keloids are itchy, hypersensitive, and prone to regrowth after they have been surgically removed. For some people who are disfigured by them, keloid scars, like proud flesh, may be a bigger problem than the initial wound was.

Even though her doctor laughed at Shannon's request for a tiny scar, scar disfigurement is a serious matter. Medically, scars from burns, extensive surgeries, and injuries are a significant focus of health care. They cause contractures, adhesions, disfigurement, and social stigma. These events limit the function of the body, cause recurrent pain, distort healthy tissue, and continually remind the person of their ongoing woundedness. Every year, over $12 billion is spent on scar treatments in the United States, and 100 million people in the developed world receive new surgical scars.[1]

Annually in the developed world, over eleven million people deal with keloid scars and four million with burn scars, most of them children and adolescents. The psychological toll can be the greatest injury. Those with facial scars often experience lifelong stigma, anxiety, and depression.[2] People with scars that result from cuts may be thought of as threatening, as the immediate assumption is that such a wound must have been caused by a violent fight.

Subconsciously, we react to people with scarred faces as villains. Think of Uncle Scar in *The Lion King*. This aversion is so widespread that there is a movement in the film industry to no longer assign facial disfigurements to malicious characters.[3] In much of the world, disfiguring scars keep people from employment, and contractures from scars leave them permanently disabled.

Various methods are used to try to revise and minimize scars that cause disability or pain. For our friends with the smaller but telltale marks of self-injury, steroid creams and injections, dermabrasions to smooth out the tissue, laser treatments, and even plastic surgeries are options. Larger scars are treated with tension-releasing dressings, gels, and scar revision surgery. Even so, the results are often not ideal.

In the case of major disfigurement, the operations needed for revisions and reshaping can go on for years.

Many people don't realize that internal scars cause problems too. Physicians refer to heart attacks as myocardial infarctions. That literally means death of heart muscle tissue. While a blocked artery may be repaired, the dead tissue in the heart typically ends up as a scar. The function of the heart is then forever changed, even if blood flow is restored. Adhesions, tight bands of scar tissue that form at the internal wound site, are complications often seen years after a surgery. Like a rope that moors a boat to a dock, the adhesions tether two internal parts of the body together, and as they tighten, they can cause bowel obstructions and other serious problems.

Regenerative medicine offers the first clear hope for permanent healing without complications from scars. Scars signify that a wound has been *repaired*, but new tissue that matches the original wounded tissue signifies that a wound has been *regenerated*. The promise of scarless healing, whether in treating burns or heart attacks, is the holy grail of wound science. It represents the ultimate goal of healing, transformation of the wound into holistic new tissue that fully conforms to the needs of the body. In some instances, it may be even better than what was there before the traumatic event.

Growth factors made by stem cells have a major role to play in regenerative medicine. They determine how rapidly the healing matrix can organize itself to better close a wound without a scar. Stem cells are simply cells that have not yet specialized—they have the ability to differentiate into various sorts of mature cell types. Though many people associate stem cells with umbilical cord blood or embryos, they are found in mature adult tissue too. In the fetus, stem cells have the potential to differentiate into any sort of cell type. As we mature outside the womb, we still have stem cells that can differentiate into specialized cell types, but their capacity for change is more restricted. For example, just as an infant can learn virtually any language at birth but is shaped to develop pathways for a certain language by being exposed to it at home, so stem cells in our bone marrow can develop into different sorts of blood cells depending on the need and the setting.

Regenerative wound science is devoted to developing methods that will remind the adult tissue of its fetal beginnings, reactivating the signals that call for rapid tissue formation just as soon as wound closure is possible. This requires a new model of that healing matrix, one that minimizes inflammation, quickens healing time, and increases relationships between many different cell types within the body, which must perform in synchrony.

☙

Perhaps in no other area of wound healing do we see such a close relationship between the physical and psychic aspects of healing. Our scars are a palpable link to past traumas and a permanent witness to both healing and suffering. Consider one character from literature who is recognized around the world by his unusual scar, which marks him as one both chosen for life and marked for death. Harry Potter's scar reminds him of things he cannot remember—the violent death of his parents, his mother's sacrifice, and the evidence of evil's powers. His scar becomes part of his identity, both to himself and to others. Strikingly, whenever there is a threat of evil in his midst, it burns with pain.[4]

More than likely we don't bear a lightning-shaped scar, and we may not even have a scar that others can see. But many of us have scars on our spirits that profoundly impact our identities as well as our roles and relationships. Our past traumas, particularly those that happened in the blurry margins of childhood, may appear like nondescript flesh wounds, but in truth, they may burn with pain whenever they are triggered by the threat of repeated harm.

As Bem and I looked anew at the science of scar formation, along with the complications and efforts at overcoming them, we saw how hypertrophic and disfiguring some of our own personal scars have been.

Bem and I grew up across the world from each other— she in the Philippines and I in the Midwest. Our languages, climates, diets, and hometown settings were nothing alike. However, we did share one thing in common so completely that once we discovered it, it was as if we'd found two identically shaped scars on our bodies. These two scars burn when in the presence of threat and contract as they mature. They may impair full function and are usually hidden in public so as to avoid judgment.

Our lives were both marked by fearful childhoods that were rich by other standards. Inside our comfortable homes, which were led by accomplished parents, mental illness and conflict reigned. The details differ, and some of our memories are hazy in the light of adulthood. However, the shape of our twin wounds is as recognizable as the scar on Harry Potter's forehead, an archetype of trauma shared by many, despite the stigma that isolates and hides it.

Bem reflects on the traumatic scarring she experienced:

I was the second child and eldest girl of six children. In our early years, my father became exhausted trying to support a large family, work hard all day in a major corporation, and deal with a wife he loved whose sanity was rapidly slipping away.

One day, he abruptly left, and we didn't see him for many days. We were hungry and had no money, so I was determined to find help. I walked to the nearest sari-sari store and asked the owner if he could give us some canned goods—corned beef, sardines, or pork and beans. I promised he would get paid. Drunk men laughed and jeered: "Inday, dili man mu-uli ang imong Papa kay buang man ang imong mama." ("Your daddy isn't coming home, little girl, because your mom is crazy.") I ignored them and looked straight at the store owner's eyes, feigning confidence and a certainty I didn't possess. Refusing to beg, I stood my ground. I would not leave until I could depart with food for my brothers and

*sisters. I succeeded. The grocer gave me the food, my
father eventually came home, and our debts were paid.*

    *A little part of my heart died that day, and like
keloid tissue, the scarring grew and spilled into healthy
areas of my life as I survived crisis after crisis. I escaped
my mother's terrifying attempts on my life and watched
my father recover from several of her knife wounds
to his face. Through countless encounters with my
mother, I always fought back—kicking, screaming, and
pushing. Just as I stood firm in that grocery store, I stood
between her and my younger siblings, never cowering.
I was the strong one, the one who would overcome and
defy these defensive wounds. I was increasingly proud of
my hardening battle scars.*

    *But by adulthood, the scars on my heart no longer
symbolized remarkable survival but instead became
constantly binding contractures to my spirit. My default
behavior was to always plan for the worst, brace for a
crisis, and prepare for repeated wounding. When my
husband became ill, I planned financial, legal, and
educational contingencies. On the outside, I looked
highly competent, able to handle anything. But on
the inside, the scars were getting thicker and tauter.*

    *Scientists have to plan for failure. My default
mechanism made sense in the lab. It allowed me to face
grant rejections and failed experiments with a stubborn
tenacity. I brought this determination to my family still
in the Philippines, helping them through the inevitable*

typhoons that destroyed their properties year after year.
I assisted in rebuilding their homes and won awards
for my laboratory discoveries. Meanwhile, scar tissue
kept advancing over the joyful parts of my inner life
each time a new crisis reinforced the rationale for my
vigilance and restraint.

Bem and I consider ourselves rational and realistic. We know that terrible things happen, medically and socially. We take pride in our resilience and perseverance through challenging careers and, in some cases, traumatic family relationships. Justice and truth matter more to us than to most. We prize clarity, a valuable asset in medical and scientific decision making. We are both used to people variously telling us we take on too much, are incredibly productive, or don't know how to relax. Many of these common attributes are, in part, the products of the common wounds we share. And several of these traits are good, as is our ultimate perspective. As Christians, we hold a final optimism, a belief that, as Julian of Norwich wrote, "All shall be well; and all shall be well; and all manner of thing shall be well."[5]

But for now, we are growing in our understanding of the ways our shared scars need revision and even transformation. In conflict, our scars can quickly contract and sear us with a hot, burning pain. We draw in tightly, tense and ready to push back to avoid reinjury. Alert, we see dangers others aren't aware of. We resist what we perceive to be a threatening show of strength by another. Like infections that prolong and distort scar formation, our histories may limit our openness to other possibilities and cause us to wrongly judge the motives of others.

Even though I swore that my own family would be one of peace and gentleness, when I feel challenged by a child's negative remark, it is easy to react reflexively with anger and opposition. Similarly, in work situations, I may take criticism as a personal attack rather than a route for improvement. My own early scars carry adhesions that pull on my sense of self, distorting my identity and often making me wonder if I will ever fully function like those without such wounded places. My childhood scar often feels full of keloid, only worsening with attempts at revision. Shame of the scar's presence has led to my covering up my difficulties, which inhibits true freedom and growth.

Fortunately, our physical body again shows us a way through this distorted landscape. Our hypertrophic and keloidal communal scars do not have to have the last word in the repair of our conflicts. Even for old familiar wounds, remodeling and revision are possible.

LIVING WITH OUR BATTLE SCARS

As we consider these ideas, an image of the resurrected Christ is worth contemplating. When Jesus appears to his disciples after his death, he invites them to touch his wounds (John 20:19-31). He is in resurrected form—he can walk through walls! Why would wounded spots, scars of a wrongful violent death, be present in a perfectly transformed body? Many wonder about this and surmise that maybe this was an intermediate sort of form taken by Jesus, one not completely restored as it would be in heaven.

None of us understand the full meaning. But clearly, Jesus wanted his disciples to know him. To trust him. To see who he really is. And to believe that those scars, which are so central to his story, are part of a claim to glory and redemption, inseparable from his restored self. That can give hope to those of us who live with scars we fear may be part of our demise, rather than part of our transformation. Life-giving revision and remodeling are more likely when we touch our collective scars, compassionately acknowledge them, and embrace the full community into the reshaping of the wound.

Compassionately trace your scars

Jesus invited his closest friends to feel the outline of his wounds. How might we better understand the scarred composition of our lives as we continue into the future? Through journaling, counseling, or small-group friendships, we can trace our own journeys. Like erecting an Ebenezer, we can discover how far we have come, noting the setbacks that seem to create contracture, adhesion, and disfigurement. We can learn that touching our scars will not destroy us but may even bring forth joy, as it did in the disciples.

Throughout my family's social isolation during the COVID-19 pandemic, we struggled to maintain a positive perspective. We became exasperated with one another as new interruptions compounded old irritations. Hypertrophy set in as tension grew. We failed, as a family, to make it through that season without creating new stresses in formerly healed relationships.

At first, I despaired. *I never should have had a family*, I thought. We weren't going to be the cheerful model for others to copy. But as I honestly shared that time with my close-knit prayer group, they touched my scars with the healing balm of their words. They encouraged me as they showed me that much had been repaired and resolved over the course of years. My counselor did the same, reminding me that these times of repeated adhesions are fewer and more infrequent than ever. Tracing my scars allowed me to see their real proportions, rather than anxiously fearing they were too large to overcome.

For larger community scars, compassionate tracing is also important. All organizations, all human gatherings, have scars if the people involved have shared life together. The danger of hypertrophy is in the overgrowth. We saw how healthy memorializing is important after initial scarring. It enables us to display the ways in which our collective scars have changed us and have redeemed some part of our life together. "We shall overcome" is a chant needed not just once, but over and over as we live together. How does the community understand its current shape in light of past wounds? How often are those scars reexamined to ensure they continue to show the best possible resolution to the past while also protecting present function?

Culturally, racial conflict has been an entrenched part of

human life. In the United States, centuries of violence against Blacks by whites and civil authorities have created a scar that has been ripped open again and again. It is so disfigured it is hard to tell where to begin making revisions that promote justice. The scar is painful to look at and acknowledge, and we naturally yearn to look away to healthier aspects of our national life. In protests right after George Floyd was killed, many people pointed out how police and authorities were kneeling in alliance with protesters, or otherwise positively pointing out a place in their community that overcame racial oppression. These actions, while well-intentioned, did not address the distorted scars. They did not validate the need for the troubled places to be seen as they had been formed and reshaped.

A quote by Persian poet Rumi speaks to this idea of compassionate tracing: "Don't turn away. Keep your gaze on the bandaged place. That's where the light enters you."[6] In these vital times, we must not turn away when our scars contract and thicken. Only by close examination will we understand how those scars fit into current functioning. Only through a collective uncovering can light penetrate the darkness. Naming, touching, and feeling the contours of our scars collectively are first steps toward knowing where revision is needed and how a healthier form may be sculpted.

Overcome stigma

Fear of judgment has a lot to do with our resistance to allowing the healthy tissue of community to tug us toward remodeling so that our scars don't become overwhelming. Jesus' scars are called *stigmata*. Though the word is just the plural form of stigma, it has been redefined for Christian use to imply a particular closeness to the heart of God. In Catholic mysticism, *stigmata* appear on the hands, feet, side, or head of a holy person as an outward evidence of divine favor. The scorn intended with the word is instead interpreted as a sign of blessing.

How we view ourselves in light of others and in light of God does affect our recovery from conflicts. In the case of physical scars, not only are some people working to end the association of scars with sinister characters; others see them as something beautiful or precious. In her international photo documentary "Behind the Scars," British journalist Sophie Mayanne portrays people with all sorts of scars. She pairs their pictures with their personal statements. Her goal is to give voice to the resilience, truth, and beauty that these people possess—not in spite of, but sometimes because of, their scars.[7]

We may not be able to make photos of our corporate scars, but we can participate in efforts to remake our interpretation of our life struggles. I am always struck by those who can politely refuse a drink with a comment that they are a recovering alcoholic. As a frequent business traveler, I know there is enormous pressure to join with colleagues over a cocktail. My own resolve at conquering habits that grip me is bolstered when I think of how transparently these folks are able to allow their scars to be aligned with their healthy selves.

The adolescents I care for have so many past traumas. While not normalizing homelessness, parental drug addiction, or family violence, our residential training center does recognize these as common experiences in the lives of our students. Our staff weave these topics into discussion groups, poster contests, and pizza nights, acknowledging the ways these events may have shaped the students. Resiliency is also celebrated, even as hardship is given voice. Decreasing the stigma of family failures increases the confidence of our young adults as they consider ways they may be better prepared for their futures.

Draw on the community

We've seen the vital role of collaboration in every phase of wound recovery. Culturally, in attending to our communal scars, we seem to rely more on outside help via individual counseling than on a pull into the embrace of community by those who are currently healthy alongside us. We meet with an intentionally disengaged therapist so we can get fixed up and then rejoin the group. Even group therapy is made up of people with similar issues and matching scars.

Of course, individual counseling and groups such as twelve-step programs are precious gifts. They provide the confidentiality and discernment in sharing that are necessary safeguards to healing. They can offer a safe space to start the long process of working through disfiguring life experiences. Like type III collagen, the individual work we do can get us ready for a phase that will include yet more change and even some death. But at some point, we have to understand as a body how to reincorporate our gathered wound edges into something that allows full inclusion and function within the whole.

As churches confront the history and the continuing presence of sexual abuse within their organizations, many who have experienced trauma have been given voices. Some of the perpetrators have been punished. Hopefully, careful therapeutic recovery has taken place. But those critical first steps are only a beginning.

With those who have been hurt, churches must consider how the wounded may be enfolded back into community. To guard against reinjury, how has the community of faith changed so that it is safe? Is there a possibility for a fully functional whole, even healthier than the original? This is what the world is looking for as it watches churches address abuse. Either the church is just another organization that needs to address corruption within it, or it really is a body, a living organism, that can and will be made whole.

In my own life, as my family scars tend toward a keloid-like overgrowth, community has shaped the revision of those scars. Through patient friendships that give time and space for the real complaint of the soul to be voiced, my wound site experiences less tension. Faithful women who gather for prayer and encouragement pull me close. My husband's words of validation act like growth factors, promoting regeneration and boosting healing time. Stretching and softening take place whenever I soak in the beauty of this magnificent world or laugh loudly with a group of friends. Understanding the image of another as a fellow wound bearer removes much of the isolating stigma. Letting go of control and just holding up a healthy vision of my family's future prevents inflammation and promotes hope for final restoration.

Bem's story is also a witness to the power of ongoing revision and transformation:

After I got married, I contemplated for many years how to avoid the possibility of being a terrible mother, or worse, passing on defective genes to my child. Pregnancy was not in my careful calculations.

As badly as my childhood had maimed my heart and mind, I felt the Lord impress me with a new understanding. Although I could have made it biologically impossible to have a child, an instinct or nudging always stopped me from choosing this permanent path. One morning after my daily Bible reading on the story of the Israelites and the Promised Land, I had a sense that God would bless Julio and me with a son someday, a "Caleb."

And so, after seven years of marriage, my son was born. My only child is named after a famous faithful warrior, a strong man, highly favored by God. Caleb is known in the Bible as a slayer of giants in the Promised Land. He was unafraid of claiming new, dangerous territory that others ran away from—unbroken by old age and years of roaming in the wilderness. My son has

*grown into a fine young adult, and in over two decades
of being his mother, I have not harmed him as I once
feared my genetic makeup might lead me to do. Being
a mother became an adventure in which healing could
be made visible, where God could work on revising the
scars of my deepest wounding.*

Our deepest wounds—in our physical bodies as well as
our corporate ones—bear witness to trauma, pain, inflammation, and distortion. Yet individually and corporately we
testify as wound bearers to the remarkable interdependent
process that propels us toward healing, resolution, and new
life. We are designed in the image of God to be oriented
toward healing. The phases of hemostasis, inflammation,
tissue formation, and remodeling guide us through the
stages required to recover from the hurtful experiences of
our human lives. Even so, there is more. Regeneration, rather
than restoration, calls us to real transformation. There we
find ultimate hope for being made new.

CHAPTER 8

IN THE BEGINNING

Innocence and Perfection

*Last of all he said, "Lucy, Eve's Daughter," and Lucy came
forward. He gave her a little bottle of what looked like glass (but
people said afterwards that it was made of diamond) and a small dagger.
"In this bottle," he said, "there is a cordial made of the juice of one of
the fire-flowers that grow on the mountains of the sun. If you or any
of your friends are hurt, a few drops of this will restore you."*
C. S. LEWIS, *The Lion, the Witch and the Wardrobe*

FINLEY'S PARENTS CUDDLE their healthy little boy, telling him
he's been born twice. They don't mean this in a religious
sense. They mean it in a physical one, and they have pictures
to prove it.

At just under twenty weeks of gestation, the halfway point
of pregnancy, Finley had surgery to repair a life-threatening
birth defect. Doctors opened his mother's womb, carefully
operating on him while keeping him tethered to his mother
by his umbilical cord. The process, called open fetal surgery, is performed by select teams of specialists to repair rare
conditions that are fatal if left untreated until natural birth
occurs. Though the procedure is risky to both mother and

fetus, success stories like Finley's drive surgeons to test the limits of medical technology as they brave new frontiers.

Such advances cause doctors and patients to marvel and celebrate the continually unfolding potential for healing through the applications of science and the human spirit. But in Finley's case, one aspect of his healing remains a mystery, even to the innovative and skilled surgeons who treated him: Finley's skin bears no scars from his surgery. In several places where his skin was cut for access to organs and then stitched back together, the only marks that could be found at birth were the stitch remnants. The medical team cannot claim responsibility for this and are amazed by it, even though they've seen it before.

The fetal surgeons speak in awe about this process, known as scarless healing. It occurs in a number of species but was first seen in humans toward the end of the twentieth century as fetal surgery was evolving. Depending on the size and location of the wound, the developing fetus tends to heal from wounds without forming scars until about twenty to twenty-four weeks gestation. Rather than replacement scar tissue forming, the existing tissue is wholly repaired—true regeneration occurs. It is as if the wound never happened.

For the past thirty years, scientists have been working hard to figure out why this is. What qualities in the fetus are lost with maturation? Harnessing this power could revolutionize wound therapy following catastrophic burns, facial deformities, and other causes of severe disfigurement made worse by contractures associated with scars.

Research continues, but scientists have identified four major differences between wound healing after birth and while in the womb. Complex interactions between the inflammatory cells, the extracellular matrix (ECM), the cell mediators, and growth factors result in very different outcomes.

The fetus has a much lower level of inflammation in response to most wounds compared to the adult. To put it in plain terms, it is less defensive. Since scars are part of the defensive reaction to wounds associated with inflammation in the immune response, early theories suggested that amniotic fluid provided a sterile environment, so the fetus didn't need to draw on its defenses. That theory was abandoned when it was pointed out that marsupials (such as the kangaroo) develop in the dirty pouches of their mothers yet also experience scarless healing in early gestation.

Fetal tissue doesn't respond as if a wound will destroy it and doesn't send out an abundance of defensive units to make sure it will stay safe from a foreign attack. It remains rather innocent—truly naive. The fetus sends just the right number of inflammatory cells to repair a clean wound. In the case of bacteria, that may not be such a good thing—we call fetuses, as well as newborns, immunocompromised. They are not good at recognizing and defending themselves against germs.

In contrast, the adult body triggers an immediate, aggressive response to an outside assault, whether it is fully needed or not. Too much defense, as we've seen, leads to unnecessary granulation and scarring. But even appropriate mature inflammation is too prolonged to result in scarless healing. The fetus seems to send out the exactly needed amount, no more and no less than required.

The next difference between wound healing in the fetus and the mature human is in the ECM. The fetal matrix almost immediately gets to work to remodel tissue, providing a sticky surface for cells to move and build upon, and generally acts like a neighborhood of Amish barn raisers who gather at sunrise. The fetal wound gets lots of early support, but the injuries experienced after birth have to wait around longer for that matrix to become helpful. The adult healing matrix readies itself when called but may hit the snooze button a time or two before rolling out of bed.

While the fetus's healing matrix is vigorous, the mediators—communicators to the inflammatory soldier cells—aren't as active as they are in adults. This also contributes to a quieter inflammatory response. In adults, on the other hand, these mediators act like memory keepers of wounds—with a subsequent strike, they are ready very quickly, increasing the inflammatory potential.

Unlike the mediators, growth factors are quickly called in during fetal wound healing. The intention is to close a wound as fast as possible without inflammation and scarring. Cell growth, true regeneration, is the focus. There is no sluggish filling of a wound that results in a slower closure with its inevitable scar. Growth is more of a prolonged journey in mature bodies, while in the developing fetus, it is primary.

Through her work, Bem has uncovered some of the mysteries of this tissue regeneration. As a young scientist working in a federal research lab, she discovered one of the proteins that sends signals for tissue growth and maturation, rather than scarring. She did so by looking for the genetic defect that prematurely interrupted this process in a group of mutant mice. This type of genetic research is how we discover much of what is necessary for healthy life—we look at mutations and learn how they interrupt a normal sequence of events. In Bem's case, she studied mice that seemed to grow perfectly as fetuses, but soon after they were born, they all died.[1]

To identify the genetic defect causing these mice to die, Bem's team sequenced and catalogued over a million base pairs of mouse DNA (the building blocks that code the gene), comparing the DNA code of healthy mice to that of the mutant ones. Another group designed a tiny micro CT scanner for the mice, allowing visualization of their organs and soft tissues. Other researchers invented ways to make the tissues transparent so they could actually see into the bones and cartilage.

Why expend such efforts on a small group of rodents? Bem realized that the disrupted gene had a very specific function. It controlled tissue growth and maturation during early development, not just in mice but also in other mammals—including humans. When this gene was disrupted, the tissues would grow to a certain point and look healthy, but they stopped developing before becoming functional mature tissue.

As it turned out, the majority of the genes affected by the mouse mutation had a special role in building tissue stability. They coded, or directed, the proteins that were part of the ECM. The ECM (extracellular matrix), you may recall, is material like biological superglue that is secreted outside the cells and acts to hold the cells together in a certain formation, like a scaffold or a 3D building framework. In addition, the ECM acts as a communication superhighway for processes in and out of the cells. In the fetus, the gene expression of this matrix is set up for very rapid tissue formation, preparing the baby for life outside the mother's womb. So the altered gene expression meant the ECM was faulty and the framework for holding together the tissues undeveloped. Everything collapsed when the fetus no longer had its mother's support.

When the gene acts as intended, it works best in fetal life and the early newborn period. Lower amounts of the protein are found as we age, which is consistent with what we know about wound healing—we get more scars and slower healing as we get older. Bem's lab is working on methods to reactivate adult tissue using the fetal protein as a signaling device. If scientists can use that protein to tell mature cells to optimize growth like the fetus does, then tissue regeneration of wounds is a real possibility.

For now, scientists haven't been able to collectively harness fetal power to change our wound-healing patterns so that scar formation is eliminated. But regenerative medicine is an expanding field, and visions of that healing elixir with powers beyond the realm of our ordinary world, like the cordial that Father Christmas gives to Lucy in *The Lion, the Witch and the Wardrobe*, spur on the science. The original created order of our human lives is quickly replaced after birth with a tougher version. Restoring the signals that would allow for tissue regeneration rather than scarring is elusive, to be undertaken with as much caution as hope.

ℭℜ

Advancements in our understanding of fetal tissue regeneration have much to teach us about healing corporate wounds. Is scarless healing a worthy pursuit in our collective life, or just the stuff of fairy tales? Could we ever respond with just the right amount of inflammation, immediate supportive collaboration, quiet purposeful mediation, and an agreement to pursue growth over division?

The idea of achieving a scar-free life does capture our imaginations. Even so, it's hard for me to visualize my physical body without them. My scars are so much a part of me. The fingers with multiple matchstick-sized mounds where warts were burned off when I was a child. My left knee with the map of South America made when my bike spun out of control in the gravel at the bottom of a hill. My right thigh with a four-inch gash from the time I was getting shots for kindergarten and moved my leg while the needle stayed in place. That was when I first said, quite fiercely, that I was going to be a doctor—not a nurse, not the one who gives shots.

Perhaps, like going back to fetal life, there is an innocence we can't recapture. The immune system gets better at recognizing threats when it has more of an exposure history. It's the same with us as we navigate our outer world. We learn to be quickly defensive after we feel we have been targeted. If trust is breached, we may decide that an aggressive initial reaction seems pretty rational. Some level of defensiveness is clearly appropriate as we strive to protect ourselves.

In fact, our repeated corporate wounds take a toll at both the molecular and the larger external level. We now understand that profound trauma actually damages our DNA, shortening our telomeres, those protective caps on the end of the strands, similar to the plastic wrappers at the ends of shoestrings. The damage contributes to chronic diseases like diabetes, arthritis, and heart disease. Adverse childhood experiences (ACEs), which include such stresses as abuse, neglect, domestic violence, or a family member's incarceration, can even affect the development of the next generation in utero, as the wound somehow becomes imprinted into the newly forming DNA.[2] Maybe this new understanding of molecular genetics helps make sense of generational curses in the Bible: Exodus 34:7 says that the iniquity of parents is laid on their children down to the third and fourth generations. That verse always seemed so unjust to me, but perhaps it is just stating a fact.

The lesson of scarless healing seems to be that the more readily available and mobilized the community is, the less defensive the injured must be, and the more easily they can move toward restoration and renewal. For many of us, this requires a cultural shift from our ideas about self-sufficiency, maturity, and independence. To receive such support, we must acknowledge our dependency and be vulnerable and open about our weakness. Trust is perhaps most important of all.

In her book *Daring Greatly*, sociologist Brené Brown writes about the transformative power of vulnerability, which is opening ourselves to others in a way that exposes us to the risk of being hurt.[3] It is a response that must be weighed, a posture that lays down many defenses. Requiring deep trust, Brown asserts that vulnerability is a necessary prerequisite for authentic connection and healthy relationships in every sphere of life. Many of us may associate vulnerability with weakness and exposure, thinking of children or refugees in perilous positions against stronger forces. But in Brown's usage, vulnerability is a conscious choice made by one who has strength.

As a pediatrician, I spend many days attending to children we label as vulnerable, unguarded, or defenseless. Usually we mean that these children need extra care, as they are at risk for harm. But often those of us who work with special-needs children find they have strengths that inspire us. Over the years, I've treated a number of patients with Down syndrome. I frequently hear others say that they are happier than most people. I haven't necessarily found this to be true, but I do think they trust easily and are open, vulnerable, and often quicker to forgive. These qualities mirror those of rapid scarless healing and may have something to do with the positive image we assign to people with Down syndrome. At the same time, they sometimes need coaching in healthy defensiveness to remain safe, as well as to learn how to set boundaries and interact with those who may take advantage of them. Even as adolescents and adults, they rely on a strong network of community support.

Brown warns that when we numb vulnerability, we also diminish positive traits such as joy, gratitude, and purpose. We seek to make the uncertain certain—no mysteries are allowed, whether in politics, religion, or my dispute with an annoying neighbor. When we assume we are always right while the other is always wrong, we shut down discourse, cutting off any opportunity for healing.[4] Getting vulnerability just right is the work of a lifetime.

The mediators—namely the cytokines and other cells that increase inflammation and self-defense—remain mostly quiet in the fetus. Remember the biblical Job's would-be mediators, who certainly didn't remain quiet as they continued to sit with him in his woundedness. Instead they accused and criticized. In times of trauma we need mediators, but ones who want to move us forward toward wholeness, not keep a festering wound open. Even when we clearly have been wronged, a good mediator acknowledges and supports the truth of that injustice, while gently assisting us so we can safely enter a place of regeneration. In doing so, the mediator seeks to limit defensiveness.

As my church engaged in a particularly long and difficult consideration of policies, we learned that some of our congregants no longer trusted the church's leadership because of their past actions. These events occurred before any current church elders were in their positions. The leaders invited the person who seemed to speak for the group to meet and air their grievances so the new board members could understand the problems. Unfortunately, the invitation was never accepted. As time went on, church policies were discussed but not established, as there was no clarity on what was needed. Treasured members of the church left rather than move into community healing. In short, the mediators had remained in defensive postures, choosing anger over vulnerability. The scars are thick.

A strong and rapid community response is the best protection against scarring. This has become clear to me in my work with many children who have gone through an ACE such as abuse or neglect. So often, the community is not there for the wounded one. Unless very severe, childhood trauma is frequently not uncovered until years later. Or when it is discovered, children must rely on a system that may constantly interrupt caregiving rather than networking it together into a seamless, coordinated whole. As a result, original traumas give way to new ones.

At my daughter's swim meet, I sat next to a friend who had welcomed a four-year-old foster child the night before. He climbed all over the bleachers, apparently in good spirits despite his new surroundings. Then when he turned to get my friend's attention, he tugged on her arm and called her Mommy. He had been in so many new settings that this name was just a label for the woman who got you up in the morning. Though he might have looked unscarred to a casual observer, his wounds were far from healed.

As we go through life, we may get the idea that our healing should be a solitary rather than a communal endeavor. American society and the health care community prize autonomy. It is so ingrained, we even reinforce it when we physicians seek to offer social support. In medical visits, we ask patients screening questions about depression, domestic violence, PTSD, and ACEs without ever asking who is there for support and what role family, friends, faith, and community play in their lives. The medical forms provide no narrative for assisting the patient unless there is a present danger—they are simply checklists so we can survey the factors that might contribute to the individual's poor health. We assume the patient somehow navigates all those issues like a pilgrim sent on a solitary quest. In the isolation of a sterile exam room, the questions alone can trigger fresh wounds, with little time allowed for a helpful response.

How can we, as members of our own communities, act more like the fetal healing matrix? I came across one powerful example in the media just as I was writing this chapter. A pregnant mother was traveling with her toddler when he had an utter meltdown in the airport boarding area. The mother sat down, put her head in her hands, and cried. Instead of ignoring or shaming her, a number of women in the boarding area quietly got up from their seats and encircled her and her child. They offered fruit and sang to the little boy, and they soothed both mother and son. Then when it was time to board, everyone got up and scattered, restored and ready to continue their journeys.[5] This is an illustration of the fetal matrix in action—quickly present, surrounding the wound, focused on providing closure, and building a scaffold for healing that is regenerative.

It contrasts with another news story I came across that same week. A man posted a video of a toddler having a tantrum on an international flight, with apparently no help given to the mother traveling alone. Nothing constructive happened on the flight. Nothing constructive came from the post either—only a barrage of destructive and mocking comments directed at the mother, her child, and the man who posted the video.[6]

Scars may be ugly, but they don't hurt much as they form. That is because most scars don't have nerves. Scarless healing, on the other hand, requires suffering. Even though inflammation can be painful as well, tissue regeneration is no easy process. New tissue is quite tender, and nothing burns more than a growing young nerve. Remodeling and final shaping require cell death as well as growth. Everything loses something in the process, just as everything gains. The final result is tissue that blends seamlessly with the original—no individuality remains, no wound site to notice and recall a past injury.

We are just on the frontier of this kind of healing in our corporate life, whether in medicine, society, or the church. Our focus still is very individual and against personal suffering. If we do turn the other cheek, we'd at least like someone to notice. Nimble communities form online with GoFundMe and other crowdfunding platforms, but coming together physically as the body of Christ gathered and given is a trickier thing. This is particularly true when we want to be responsive not just to social needs but to complex wounds. Suffering, individually and as a community, is not usually our desired first option on the road to healing. Persecuted churches across the world may have more ready illustrations than we in the First World do.

In America, and across the globe, there are increasing calls for racial regeneration—for an entirely new way of looking at the social body of our lives together as people of diverse ethnicities and backgrounds. The protests against racism aren't new—they have been ongoing in the United States since the times of slavery. Abolition didn't heal the wounds of racism. Neither did Reconstruction or the civil rights movement. As a popular social media message notes, "Racism is the wound America never properly treated. Now that wound is infected." Joe Biden put it in a way more in keeping with our metaphor: "It's time for us to face the deep, open wound of systemic racism. . . . Nothing about this is going to be easy or comfortable, but if we simply allow this wound to scab over once more without treating the underlying injury, we'll never truly heal."[7]

Overcoming racism necessitates more than reforms. It requires new hearts. Racial regeneration certainly is in line with the gospel—a kingdom where there is no Jew or

Gentile, no slave or free, no male or female—and yet where each person is treasured as unique, individual, and made in the image of God.[8] Howard Thurman, an African American theologian, scholar, and civil rights activist, understood that our corporate body would need to undergo transformation for lasting health to be possible. Raised by his grandmother, a former slave, Thurman cofounded the first US interracial, multiethnic church, Church for the Fellowship of All Peoples in San Francisco.[9] As Thurman matured, he saw the need for new growth to promote a body of Christ that was inclusive and beautiful in its diversity, but unified as a whole.

In his book *Jesus and the Disinherited*, Thurman calls people to loving, nonviolent action against injustice, which has to start with self-denial of hatred toward oppressors. Reflecting on his life's work in *Footprints of a Dream*, he shares: "The movement of the Spirit of God in the hearts of men often calls them to act against the spirit of their times, or causes them to anticipate a spirit which is yet in the making. In a moment of dedication, they are given wisdom and courage to dare a deed that challenges and to kindle a hope that inspires."[10]

It's not clear from our history that we would necessarily choose scarless healing if given the chance. The prototypical first humans, Adam and Eve, chose wound upon wound. First was the trespass of taking what did not belong to them. Lies followed. With the loss of innocence and the knowledge of good and evil came defensiveness. The serpent made me! She gave it to me! The blame was always on another. Flares of defensiveness prevailed until Adam and Eve encapsulated themselves in clothing made of fig leaves, trying to become invulnerable and showing they were no longer one with the community. They were then driven out of the Garden, in isolation and apart from any restoration of the original organic whole, that good creation as it was meant to be. The wound would stay open as original sin, a reminder to all of the first corporate wound.

So while scarless healing may be possible through regenerative medicine, it seems an idealistic reach in the world of broken relationships and accumulated hurts. Minimum defensiveness, healthy communities ready to serve, clean wound margins, and a relentless pursuit of growth and transformation are lofty aspirations. What should we hope for? After all, even Jesus appeared with clear evidence of his wounds after his resurrection.

We hear the phrase *forgive and forget*. Is this a picture of scarless healing? Unfortunately, this statement has been used to deny the reality of the wound, to ask the victim to cover up a trauma and then hold it in secret if it can't truly be forgotten. Certainly, this isn't healthy healing. Yet we hear that as far as the east is from the west, so far has God removed our sins against him (see Psalm 103:12). Is it possible to forgive so well that we truly can emotionally forget holding the offense against the perpetrator? Can we embark on a wholly restored relationship, even when the injury has been serious? Powerful examples do give us hope, as we look at the lives of Corrie ten Boom and Nelson Mandela. And consider Dorothy Holloway. After her son was murdered, this Arkansas resident descended into a pit of grief and despair. Eventually, though, she realized she needed to forgive the man who'd killed him. When she sent the convicted prisoner a letter, she had no idea how guilty he felt and how much he wanted her absolution. Soon she had not only forgiven the murderer of her child but also entered into a loving friendship with him.[11] She showed remarkable trust, vulnerability, openness, and a willingness to encounter further suffering in the cause of more perfect healing.

There's another story in the Bible, one that beckons a new Eden. The Gospels tell us that on a certain Sabbath day, Jesus was teaching in the synagogue. He knew that the religious elite there were watching to see if he would perform a healing miracle so they could accuse him of working on the Sabbath. Jesus responded by asking a man, whose right hand was shriveled, to stand before everyone and stretch out his hand. After the man complied, his hand was made fully new (see Luke 6:6-10).

The reasons behind this miracle of Jesus are not completely known, but some of the details are instructive. The Sabbath is the crowning day of all creation—the day when humans, the earth, all its creatures, and God are meant to be in perfect harmony, a state of shalom. The traditional Jewish greeting "Shabbat shalom" symbolizes the perfection seen in the celebration of this day. It is a symbol of fullness, of completion. Rather than allowing the evil of impairment to persist into this space, Jesus taught that it was good to seek wholeness over traditions that cripple.

Tradition has it that Luke was a physician, and it is noteworthy that he alone specifies that it was the man's right hand that was disfigured. In that time, and even today in much of the Eastern world, the right hand is considered honorable and the left hand untouchable. Eating, greeting, and writing are all done with the right hand. I saw this firsthand when treating patients in India. The withering of a right hand would have impaired a person's ability to thrive in numerous cultural settings.

When Jesus heals this man's hand, it is as if he gives him a new birth. His body is now whole. It is an image of resurrection, of being complete as we were intended. As for how Jesus did it, we call it a miracle. But it's reasonable to believe that Jesus harnessed the very processes at work in fetal healing—just at a supernatural pace. The idea gives me hope for glimpses of such healing in our social lives.

Some people point to the reality of their scars in this place and time as tools for growth. It's not that they would choose the wounds. But the visible signs of cancer surgery, a trauma survived, or an amputated limb remind them of where they have been and who has been with them. They identify with those who suffer, as they, too, have suffered. Their scars tell stories not so much of failing but of overcoming. Perhaps that is also a sign of regenerative healing.

We all wonder what life was meant to be like, what perfection really looks like. We live in a state that is often referred to by Christians as "already but not yet." This isn't Eden. It isn't heaven. We do have scars and visible wounds. But just because Jesus used his wounds to show it was really he who suffered doesn't mean that his own ultimate regeneration includes scars. His healing miracles raised the dead, restored sight, allowed the lame to walk, and in many ways gave new life to those who knew only the deep wounds of a broken world. So much is still a mystery. All we know is what we yearn for. And so we reach for those places where we can trust more, open ourselves up, join community, suffer for the sake of healing, and participate in unexpectedly wondrous new growth.

CHAPTER 9

MIND AND BODY AS ONE

Science, Spirituality, and Transformation

*Love protects us from nothing, even as it
unexplainably sustains us in all things.*

JAMES FINLEY

SHORTLY AFTER MY FAMILY MOVED to Washington State from
North Carolina, I received a phone call from a physician
friend who also worked in migrant health. His tone was
urgent. He asked if I knew a local *curandero*, a traditional
healer who works with Mexican and indigenous peoples
of Latin America. A baby in critical condition was being
treated in a Seattle hospital, and the family insisted that one
be brought to the room. The infant was not expected to live,
and the family did not believe that all was being done to save
the infant's life in the absence of a *curandero*. The hospital
had never worked with a *curandero* before and had no idea
how to find one. My friend had been contacted as calls went
out to anyone who might be able to help this family.

Thankfully, a *curandero* was located rather quickly, and amazingly, the hospital set aside its restrictions to allow traditional healing practices in the sterile hospital room filled with modern machinery. The *curandero* entered with a collection of leafy branches, a small mortar and pestle, religious candles, and paper bags filled with herbs. The candles were lit, prayers were said with the family, and then the child was swept with the branches, gentle rhythmic motions down each side of her body, just grazing her skin. Herbs were ground into a paste. A handmade cigarette stuffed with some sort of dried herb was lit, inhaled by the *curandero* and then exhaled in a sweet pungent haze over the child. Some of the cigarette must have been chewed because the *curandero* intermittently made a few forceful spits in the direction of the child's chest. Prayers and chanting in Spanish continued, with all present circling the bed. The family wept, knowing that their child had at last received comprehensive care in her fight for life.

Though US physicians are often ignorant of *curanderos'* practices, an estimated 25 percent of Mexican immigrants, particularly those who'd recently arrived from rural locations, use them as an adjunct to the health care they receive from licensed providers.[1] *Curanderismo*, the practice of healing performed by these men and women, is an amalgamation of herbal medicine, spiritual and religious practices, massage, counseling, cultural rituals, and Western medicine. *Curanderos* may do everything from injecting antibiotics for presumed infections to casting out an evil spirit causing chronic pain. They are believed to have special healing gifts

bestowed by God, and they see their work as a true vocation. Typically, they earn a living through gifts and donations
rather than by charging for their compassionate care.[2]

Early in my work in migrant health, I realized that many
of the methods I'd been taught were not trusted by my immigrant patients. Dispassionate objective care needed to be set
aside initially. Efficiency was not a value. These patients
expected to engage in informal conversation with me before
I was to begin my inquiry into the patient's presenting problem. *Personalismo* mattered as much as the correct diagnosis. How was my family? What grades were my children in?
Where did my parents live? Did I go to church? My own life,
as well as my patient's particular life story, had to be understood. No rushing.

If our patients thought we didn't listen and understand,
they were more likely to seek other ways of healing. *Curanderos*
are technically lay healers, known in the cultural community
but hidden from the wider world. Our patients used them
for everything from providing Depo-Provera shots for birth
control to offering marriage counseling to treating *nervios*.
(*Nervios* is a condition much akin to PTSD and a common
malady in struggling immigrants who have fled violence and
terror but find themselves unwelcome and alone in their new
setting.) Acknowledging the use of *curanderos* was important
as I collaborated with our patients in their healing.

In medical school, practices such as *curanderismo* were
referred to as folk medicine. The implication was that
it was quackery, a primitive use of magic and religious

appropriations. It belonged to those who had no other choices in health care, and it was said to have no evidence base to support its usefulness. Acupuncture, massage, and naturopathy received slightly better reviews, but all were believed unnecessary in the light of the rigorous science assumed to support our own education and practices.

One important aspect of the practices that were marginalized during my education is that they do not harbor a mind-body distinction. That is, they see no dichotomy between physical ailments and psychic or spiritual suffering. Mind, body, and spirit are viewed as one, so the role of each in healing is acknowledged. This outlook is mostly absent from standard medical texts and practice.

While I didn't grow up with *curanderos*, I did grow up with religious rituals that connected the body to the spirit and were believed to promote health. Each February, I lined up with my Catholic schoolmates so the local priest could bless my throat. This was done to honor the Feast of St. Blaise, the patron saint of sore throats. I always wondered, more curious than skeptical, how much strep throat was prevented through these exercises.

My husband remembers a different ritual in his small North Carolina hometown. His father, a family doctor, would often be asked to remove a wart. The standard treatment then was to cauterize the wart, burning the flesh. If the wart came back, his father summoned the office nurse, Edith, to the exam room. She was considered a specialist in the removal of difficult warts. She sat with the patient and "prayed it away." Over and over again, patients would proclaim that Edith had cured their warts. Evidently, her ability was confined to warts; as far as my husband recalls, she wasn't enlisted to help eliminate other disorders.

As a matter of fact, there is a robust medical anthropology associated with warts. For centuries, wart healers and wart removal practices have been codified into the norms of health care. Such widespread belief in the power of prayer to remove warts persists that randomized-controlled studies have been undertaken to measure its effectiveness. These studies were done using prayers consistent with the warty patient's religious identity—Muslim, Christian, or Buddhist. What worked? It depends on how you ask the question. There was no difference in wart elimination between groups that received prayer and those that did not. But there *was* a difference between those participants who believed in the power of the prayer and those who did not. Those who did tended to have warts eradicated more quickly than those who did not trust the power of either the intercessor or the prayer itself.[3]

Prayer, of course, has long been associated with healing. Typically, it is thought of as independent of the biochemical healing mechanism, acting as a "ghost in the machine." Prayer transcends culture and even belief. An atheist may remark that she will "think" of a friend as that friend undergoes surgery. Whether thinking positive thoughts, or reciting an intercessory prayer, people offer up their own intentions with some faith in the power of these practices to assist recovery from disease.

Conventional Western medicine centers on treatments for the physical body when addressing a particular disease or health problem. Complementary and alternative medicine (CAM), on the other hand, is more holistic and treatments often involve the body, mind, and spirit. Acupuncture, massage, healing prayer, herbal medicine, Reiki, and more are some of the practices used in CAM. There are typically three responses to this form of medicine. It may be dismissed as quackery and seen as totally ineffective other than providing a placebo effect. Or it may be met with skepticism as well as some measure of openness to a poorly understood nonscientific effect. Finally, it may be embraced as a powerful and productive medical tool, in many ways superior to a "toxic" Western model. Those who dismiss CAM and those who wholeheartedly endorse it rarely agree on a set of therapies that might integrate their separate views. Those in the middle group lack experience with CAM but are curious about how it may work, wanting to avoid harm while maximizing good. In some ways, the mind-body dualism still triumphs in all three responses—the body's healing mechanisms are either biochemically and unconsciously driven, or they respond to intentional thoughts and practices that are rooted in the psyche. For example, while surgery and yoga may both be advised for the repair of a hip, it is rare to see a discussion of the interplay between the biochemical processes of wound healing and the mindful techniques that are components of yoga.

How does any of this relate to the four phases of wound

healing? It turns out that the mind and body are indeed unified and that our thoughts and feelings have a lot to do with
the activation of our wound-healing chemicals. In her book
Cure: A Journey into the Science of Mind Over Body, author
Jo Marchant examines the science behind healing associated
with such things as prayer, energy fields, and placebo effects.[4]
Marchant is herself a scientist, motivated to write the book
to record her study of how physical processes are affected by
states of the mind.

Marchant discusses the placebo effect in depth. A placebo
is defined as an inert substance or harmless medical technique that offers no proven benefit but is sometimes used as
a method of fooling patients into thinking they are getting
some sort of therapy. When new pharmaceutical drugs are
being tested for effectiveness, they are tested against place-
bos. Ideally, this testing happens in a double-blind randomized controlled trial. This means that the researcher giving
the medicine and the person receiving it don't know if the
substance offered is the new drug or the placebo—they are
"double-blinded." Further, the people in the trial are randomly sorted into the placebo group and the "real" drug
group—they are "randomly controlled" to avoid bias. These
careful considerations are meant to remove any possibility
that something other than the effectiveness of the pharmaceutical could affect the results.

During these trials, people in the placebo group commonly show some improvement in their symptoms. They
may even claim persistent relief from their disease. This is

referred to as the placebo effect. Just believing that one is getting a beneficial treatment seems to help relieve distress. Commonly, the placebo effect is relegated to the sidelines, seen as a side effect of wishful thinking, a product of the mind tricking us. We are easily fooled, say the experts. When a trial drug has the same effect as the placebo, both are discarded as useless, even if both groups showed measurable improvement.

Early in a new health crisis, incompletely tested methods may be given as emergency efforts to help patients who seem to have no options left for care. But as time goes on, researchers try to set up tests of treatments that will yield results that can be widely trusted as a direct result of the new therapy. For instance, we saw many people defend the role of placebo-controlled trials for treatments of COVID-19. But before long, some popularized medications used to treat this virus were sidelined because scientists weren't confident that the medication was more beneficial than the placebo. In other words, the apparent positive effects noted in early treatment may have simply been placebo effects. Bias, as well as placebo, may have promoted initial belief in the drugs' effectiveness.

This limited understanding of the placebo effect as simply a false hope is slowly changing. Advances in measuring substances like neuropeptides (small protein-like molecules that are transmitted from our brain cells) show that our body has a signaling system that includes not just the immune system, but also the nervous system and endocrine system.

The relatively new fields of psychoneuroimmunology and psychoneuroendocrinology formally join together the mind-body separation as they examine how emotions, thoughts, and beliefs impact neuropeptide release that, in turn, sends signals to hormonal and immune centers of the body, eventually causing a direct biochemical effect on the phases of wound healing.

In other words, the placebo effect is not all in our heads. Many people have heard of the "runner's high"—the euphoric feeling one gets after running some distance, despite the hard work and stress on the body. This effect is caused, at least in part, by the release of endorphins from the brain. Endorphins are released by our pituitary gland in response to experiences like pain, stress, eating chocolate, and sexual pleasure. If that seems like a weird mix, remember that all these things involve a heightened sensory response.

The endorphins bind to our body's natural opiate receptors, so if there is pain, it is diminished with this binding. Morphine, given by physicians to dull severe pain, binds to the same sites as our natural endorphins. Though we can build up a resistance to morphine, that doesn't happen with our natural endorphins.

Evidently, placebo painkillers can also stimulate the release of endorphins. How? Our nervous system responds to the simple action of taking a pill intended to comfort us with a signal to release endorphins. The naturally occurring endorphins bind to the body's opiate receptors and do, in fact, reduce the impact of pain and aid in wound repair.

The reduction of pain by the placebo isn't "imaginary" unless one agrees that imagination causes biochemical responses that interact with our body's healing mechanisms. Pairing a placebo with a potent medication can actually condition the brain to respond to the placebo alone. Eventually our immune system responds to the placebo regardless of our belief in the drug.[5] No imagination is required.

These findings are still in trial stages, but they do give us new insight into interactions between our thoughts, environment, and physical makeup. In some ways, our growing understandings of the linkages between psychology, spirituality, endocrinology, and immunology create more questions than they answer. Why is there a blunted response from the placebo rather than a full healing response? Why are there individual variations? What about the idea of nonlocal healing—such as the healing attributed to intercessory prayer that may occur far from the ill patient?

Much of the healing process remains a mystery, but scientists do agree on a growing number of relationships between physical and psychic healing. The role of stress in impairing wound healing is well known, as we briefly reviewed in our discussion of chronic inflammation. Pain, isolation, fear, depression, and anger also slow down physical healing. How?

Three systems in our body respond to negative experiences in discreet ways, both biochemically and behaviorally. As far as the body is concerned, any negative event is perceived as a stress to well-being, whether that event is emotional or physical. The three regions of stress response are the immune system, the psychological feedback system, and the nervous system.[6] Formally, they are described as a hypothalamic pathway, a behavioral pathway, and a sympathetic nervous system pathway (see diagram below). Each path can increase the effects of the other two paths.

The hypothalamic pathway consists of the hypothalamus and pituitary, brain centers responsible for much of our hormonal stability. The secretion of the natural steroid hormone cortisol increases under stress because our body is trying to give us a burst of energy to escape danger. Prolonged release of cortisol, however, hurts our immune system. Healing is then slowed and we are prone to chronic wounds.

STRESS EFFECTS AND WOUND HEALING

IMMUNE RESPONSE	PSYCHOLOGICAL RESPONSE	NERVOUS SYSTEM RESPONSE
HYPOTHALAMIC PATHWAY Glucocorticoids and cortisol: steroid hormones reduce inflammation but also can decrease immune function	BEHAVIORAL PATHWAY Psychological behaviors: alcohol use; poor diet, sleep, and exercise; depression; anxiety	SYMPATHETIC PATHWAY Norepinephrine and epinephrine rise; adrenaline surges; hyperglycemia (high blood sugar) results

IMPAIRED WOUND HEALING

Psychological behaviors in response to stress are often intended to numb our perceptions of threat. We sleep more, eat for comfort, overmedicate pain, drink alcohol to excess, or withdraw. These behaviors can also change our hypothalamic secretions, as our body senses that our balance is out of control. In an effort to help, more cortisol is released, further damaging our immune system.

The third pathway, the sympathetic nervous system, has a curious name. It is sympathetic in the sense that it is the portion of our nervous system that responds to stress. Run! Fight! Whichever response we choose, we need bursts of energy to keep going. The sympathetic nervous system releases adrenaline when we are under stress to give us extra momentary energy. When this happens, the liver also releases glucose, our quick fuel. The problem is, chronic stress persistently raises our glucose, or blood sugar. We force our pancreas to work harder than it should and risk diabetes. We feel hungry more often and overeat. Meanwhile, the release of cortisol also affects our blood sugar and appetite, and we find ourselves becoming less healthy in almost every way. Heart disease, diabetes, stroke, and cancer all are linked to the destructive cycles of chronic stress.

As scientists and medical professionals have investigated the negative effects of stress and emotion on wound healing, they have also tried to determine ways to counter those stresses. Mindfulness, positive visualization, music, hope, and affirmations have been not just suggested but also tested for their impact on healing. Motivation to heal and to hope for the future are shown to improve healing, and many of us have anecdotal stories to support this. A dear friend of mine with late-stage cancer, for example, lived to see his daughters graduate and his eldest marry. Of course, other biological processes and factors are at work, and sometimes patients who've determined to hang on for special family events don't make it—despite holding on to hope until the end.

Social support has the strongest impact on healing of any psychological factor. Not only does our body heal through multiple community networks at a molecular level, it also relies on community networks at a personal level. Researchers have repeatedly found that those with strong social supports heal more quickly from burns, surgical wounds, heart attacks, and other serious diseases. But scientists didn't know the precise mechanism behind this or whether it alone was a determining factor in healing. Does social support just give us better motivation or hope? Can it be that perhaps patients are forced into therapy more regularly by their loved ones? No, at least that is not the complete reason. We can thank a group of hamsters for showing us that social support is itself a healing balm.

Scientists knew that they couldn't conduct a double-blind randomized control experiment with humans to discover the relationship of healing to social support. After all, it's hard to imagine withdrawing social support from people so researchers could compare them to another group with strong social support. So scientists looked to another mammal with strong social connections—the Siberian hamster.

Siberian hamsters live in community and form social bonds. In the study, when a hamster received a surgical wound and stayed in community, its stress hormone level—cortisol—was much lower than when it was isolated. The stress of the injury didn't impair wound healing for the hamster living in a social setting. More significantly, the hormone oxytocin was released in the socially housed hamsters but not in the isolated ones. Oxytocin counters the effects of cortisol released during stress. To see just how strong an effect the oxytocin had, the isolated hamsters were then injected with oxytocin. Their healing rapidly improved, and their cortisol levels decreased. Conversely, when oxytocin was blocked in the socially housed hamsters, their rate of healing slowed despite their social situation.[7]

So, what does oxytocin mean to us in human life? What is the link between social relationships and oxytocin? Some people refer to oxytocin as the "love hormone" or a "cuddle hormone." Its secretion increases when we fall head over heels in love, but also when we simply enjoy the company of others. It counters the negative effects of cortisol as it soothes us from stressful responses, decreasing perceptions of fear and anxiety. Though no diseases are linked to a deficiency in oxytocin, our understanding of this hormone does generate concerns about the isolated elderly, the use of solitary confinement, and the potentially debilitating effects of loneliness. Clinical trials are being designed to test it as a treatment for a number of mental health problems, but the complexity of the molecule and its many effects in the body make packaging it into a medication very difficult.

My own experience with oxytocin wasn't a warm and fuzzy one. Oxytocin, or Pitocin as it is known in its manufactured form, induces labor. Four of my five children were born after Pitocin jump-started my contractions. But oxytocin is also released in the process of breastfeeding, as we bond with our babies and feel that surge of mother-lion instinct to protect our vulnerable newborns.

As we consider all these mind-body connections at the biochemical levels of wound healing, should we add a fifth phase—something about the mind—to our neatly ordered four phases of hemostasis, inflammation, regeneration, and remodeling? It would be tricky to come up with a name for it, though. The psycho-neuro-immune response phase? But no, this mind-body response isn't really a phase, for it permeates the whole process. All biological processes are interrelated and interdependent. Just as the healing matrix responds to the local situation with adjustments in support, so our brain, nerves, endocrine system, and immune system spontaneously respond and form connections as situations arise that demand attention.[8]

Medical models of healing continue to expand and grow more nuanced, more complex, and still more intriguing. Harnessing not just the individual power of hope, but also the collective power of love, moves us beyond technique to interactions not directly under our control. To allow social support to shape healing is to allow idiosyncratic and possibly intrusive dynamics into our well-ordered and antiseptic world of medicine. Whether with a *curandero* or a healing prayer team, we are learning to make more room as we collaborate together as healers. Mystery will remain, even as we better understand the roles of our biochemical pathways and their response to our minds and spirits.

CR

Transformation, rather than simple restoration, is the ultimate goal of healing. A powerful image of the difference between the two is seen in attempts to respond to opiate addiction. Narcan, a medicine given in the event of an overdose, blocks the potentially deadly effects of opioids and restores breathing, circulation, and bodily function. But it doesn't do a thing for addiction. Full recovery requires multiple interrelated processes in mind, body, and spirit. Similarly, true healing from our social wounds doesn't lead to a simple return to our previous way of relating. *In social healing, deep transformation of relationships must take place. We change our minds about each other and ourselves.*

Just as it has been shown to support physical healing, so social support is key in transforming community health. One initiative is changing the way we think of social trauma and linking it with the physical health of communities. Termed the Self-Healing Communities Model and sponsored by the Robert Wood Johnson Foundation, this approach is described as "a transformational process model for improving intergenerational health."[9] It hopes to address the root causes of social problems in practical ways that draw on community leadership and involvement.

One example of this work is seen in Cowlitz County,

Washington. In 2005, leaders launched an initiative to improve living conditions in the neighborhood with the highest rate of emergency calls. A project coordinator who talked with as many residents as she could was warned repeatedly of how dangerous the streets were at night. In fact, the area was very dark, and a pack of feral dogs ran freely after sundown. While many assumed residents liked the dark because it hid illegal activity, the coordinator discovered that the real reason for the darkness was that people couldn't afford light bulbs. With the help of area civic clubs, light bulbs were provided to everyone who needed them, and a special event called Take Back the Light was planned. On the appointed evening, the neighborhood's residents all turned on their porch lights at the same time, which was also the signal for the start of a community barbecue, featuring free food and music.[10] This one small improvement—lighting at night—helped establish a culture of health in the community and led to other initiatives. The Self-Healing Communities Model certainly mirrors the body's wound-healing system, with diverse interrelationships and empowering hope emerging as pragmatic change occurs.

Homeboy Industries, based in Los Angeles, also puts flesh on these concepts. The largest gang intervention, rehabilitation, and reentry program in the world, the organization was started by a parish priest, Father Greg Boyle, in the poorest section of the city in 1986. He saw gang violence as due to "a lethal absence of hope."[11] Boyle believed that incarceration, lack of education, and the stresses of immigration left the community isolated and disconnected. He saw that members look at those outside their gangs with the attitude, *This person does not belong to me.* To address this, Homeboy Industries developed a radical model of "kinship," affirming that we all belong to each other as members of one body. Based on the theological understandings of the body of Christ and the image of God in all people, Father Boyle asks, "How do we arrive at the moment where nothing keeps us from one another?" He asserts that if kinship were a goal we all embraced, we would be celebrating peace and justice rather than still striving for it.[12]

Homeboy Industries is successfully transforming the lives of gang members and helping reduce community violence. Kinship is becoming real in the community, expressed through principles of inclusion, nonviolence, unconditional loving-kindness, and compassionate acceptance. The example of Jesus, reflects Boyle, was "to stand in the right place—not to take the right stand."[13] Thousands of former gang members have found family, education, work, and new life through this mission of inclusion and the reimagination of identity. First, though, it depended on the vision of one person seeing another in a new light.

Spiritual traditions across the world emphasize the importance of renewing our minds through mindfulness. It is a common aspect of many religions and philosophies, used in secular settings by therapists, career coaches, and fitness trainers. To be mindful is to keep one's focus on what our senses are telling us in the current moment. Being honestly present to ourselves and to each other is indeed critical for overcoming distress. Homeboys promotes mindfulness as it helps gang members stop cycles of violence and live into the idea of being related to the person standing next to you. But if we stop at mindfulness, we may have restoration without transformation.

Undergirding individual mindfulness lies the core identity that one claims. How does being mindful allow us to move to a deeper transformative healing? Christian theology integrates the renewing of the mind with the transformation of our life, and ultimately, of the world. The communal concepts of the Trinity and the body of Christ are central to fully flourishing in a wounded world and are embraced as we are called to live in community with God, the world, and each other.

Though most practical Christian teaching seems centered on knowing Jesus, we can't really know our Christian identity fully until we know Jesus in the context of the Triune God. Becoming mindful of our connection to a God who exists always in community, as well as our own mystical integration into the body of Christ, changes our responses rooted in individualism to responses that are always inclusive of their relation to their neighbors. Though it will forever be a sacred mystery too profound for our articulation, leaning into the embrace of the Trinity can transform our self-understanding from individual, struggling Jesus-followers to communal members of the holy family.

This shift in core identity took me by surprise. When I first entered the door of Christianity as an adult, I came in stumbling. I was exhausted, sad, and aching for truth. Because I had never taken a serious look at Scripture, I decided to read the Gospel of Matthew. I knew that it was the start of the New Testament, and I'd never actually read it on my own.

I was surprised to find a Jesus who spoke with authority, kindness, love—and truth. The eleventh chapter gripped me as I identified with this invitation: "Come to me, all you who are weary and burdened, and I will give you rest. Take my yoke upon you and learn from me, for I am gentle and humble in heart, and you will find rest for your souls" (Matthew 11:28-29, NIV). Years earlier, when I had run away from home and called out to God in desperation, I had heard these same words in the solitude of that night. I didn't recognize then that they were words from a Gospel. I just heard them as soothing, and I leaned into them and slept deeply, feeling embraced.

Those who suffer find rest for their weary souls. I saw that as a core part of my identity within the Christian faith. I recognized myself as a rescued victim, a survivor who was now going to live in a new land of my choosing. That seemed like enough, and so I planned to live my life in gratitude to that Savior Jesus. But I didn't understand that what I had discovered was just my initial status, not really a long-term understanding of my entire identity. It was like the condition reported on an entrance physical exam—burdened, with a good measure of sadness.

I had had plenty of catechism. In theory, I knew the

teachings about Jesus being our brother and God our Father. Somehow those two are one. It's pretty confusing, especially when you add in the Holy Spirit! I remember listening to how people prayed so I could figure out which of the three persons in one God should get called upon. And then, to make things more complex, we are told we are also in *them*. Could it get any more mystical? My mind was renewed, but it still didn't grasp much.

But one day, I experienced a transformation. The words of another Scripture passage suddenly made sense in a powerful new way: "What great love the Father has lavished on us, that we should be called children of God! And that is what we are!" (1 John 3:1, NIV). These words were written by the disciple John, known as the one Jesus loved.[14] It seems like a pretentious title, given that Jesus loves everyone. It even made me resent John a bit. Then I saw that John had another title, one that the disciples used—Son of Thunder.[15] He was a loud-mouthed guy who jockeyed for the best position at Jesus' table. Jesus never called him his best friend. It is John who called himself that after being transformed by Jesus' life, death, and resurrection.

John's entire identity changed because of Christ's love. He became the writer of the Gospel inviting the whole world into relationship with this God. He wrote books on love. He saw visions of a redeemed universe. He encountered the Trinity.[16]

Realizing that I was known by God not primarily as a survivor or as an earnest follower but as a fully loved child,

dancing with his fully loved Son and fully loved Spirit, radically changed my self-identity. Like the Celtic dances I enjoy,
I pictured myself grasping arms in and out of a holy *ceilidh*
that linked us all together. All of humanity could join in as
we were related to one another at the most profound level.

Whether through Father Boyle's kinship claims or by
our own renewed hopes in healing from family traumas,
the power of being known as integral members of an eter-
nally loving community fundamentally alters our connections with our wounded pasts. What once were known as
destructive bonds are regenerated, redemptively incorporated
into unbroken loving unity. Rather than seeing ourselves
as victims or even as survivors, we know ourselves as children of God, brothers and sisters in Christ, valued beyond
comprehension and capable of participating in the renewal
of all things. Reconciliation is the natural outflowing of
such a stance, as is written, "The old has gone, the new is
here! All of this is from God, who reconciled us to himself
through Christ and gave us the ministry of reconciliation"
(2 Corinthians 5:17-18, NIV).

Regeneration in physical wounds literally means fully
formed new tissue. Regeneration in Christian theology
means being born anew—not repaired from our wounds,
but newly made, without scars. It is evocative of fetal scarless
healing. If we really understood the power of this theological
idea, we would echo Father Boyle's words—we would be *celebrating* peace and justice rather than striving for it.

Much is made of our identity as determined by DNA

analysis. Commercials portray people who happily announce they are related to royalty or have found ancestors in far-flung places, simply by swabbing the insides of their cheeks for a chromosome test. What had been mundane in their existence is now seemingly significant. In reality, the story of one's DNA may hold a much gloomier tale. As a geneticist, Bem meets regularly with students who are terrified of being branded by their genetic codes, wondering if they are forever destined to lives of mental illness, anger, or addiction.

Here again, we see that even our brain structure and function may adapt to our patterns of thinking. As we noted in chapter 8, profound trauma and chronic stress shorten telomeres, the protective caps at the end of chromosomes. Shorter telomeres are associated with many chronic diseases, while longer telomeres are associated with longevity. Our DNA is not expressed robotically, but is responsive to many complex features, some of which are shaped by our environments. Developing a mind grounded in love, joy, peace, patience, kindness, goodness, and self-control is not only a biblical injunction, it is a life-altering pathway.[17]

However, we live in the "already but not yet" world, and we do still struggle and strain to make real the identity we long to live out. Some lessons from the way our body responds to wounds are again instructive. A new perspective on identity requires social support. The love of others both inside and outside our faith traditions can assist us. Mental and emotional debris needs to be cleared away from our long-term wounds. Negative understandings have to be replaced with positive and hopeful ideas about who we are and what the future may hold. These concepts need constant reinforcement so that healthy patterns can be set as we respond over and over to our challenges in light of our new identities.

A prominent Christian philosophy professor illustrates how this patient renewal of the mind helped him overcome debilitating anxiety and depression. In his book, *Finding Quiet*, J. P. Moreland shares how establishing new patterns of thought helped his brain, heart, and nervous system to alter destructive pathways and form healthy habitual responses to stress.[18] When he speaks of "the heart," he means all of the qualities of the mind, will, and emotions. He imagines all the organs in the body as having grooves that have been worn deep inside us by our constant patterns of behavior. Turning away from negativity and discord, and turning toward joy and peace, allows the formation of new grooves, or new pathways for health. Moreland affirms the use of medicine, counseling, and mindfulness in addition to spiritual disciplines such as prayer, Scripture study, and fasting.

Though the idea of grooves in our organs is a fanciful one, Moreland's concepts support the mind-body pathways we have examined. Joy and peace actually have biochemical properties as well as abstract ones. Optimism, social support, hope, and motivation all decrease our cortisol levels and potentially increase our oxytocin secretion. These are typically background mechanisms, operating without our expressed attention to their release. But when we shift control of our overt actions, we exert new control over our more hidden patterns. Like any regular exercise, consistency and practice are necessary for lasting change to emerge.

How can we begin to cross what may be a painful divide with those who have hurt us? Sometimes we need to harness a placebo effect. During a stressful time in my marriage, it seemed my husband and I were at an impasse. Each time one of us spoke to the other about our feelings, tensions escalated. Then our counselor told us to try a placebo.

He didn't actually use those words. Instead, he asked us to each make a list of all the things we enjoyed when we were dating. What were all the little things one person did or said to encourage the other? We were to share our lists with each other and then practice doing those things again. He told us it was fine if, at first, our efforts seemed fake. The point was to actually do the kind thing, realizing that the other person would appreciate it.

Our counselor was right. Even though we knew they were acts of the will rather than emotions, over time those little habits took root and became real impulses. Loving empathy and goodwill returned. New and deeper grooves were formed, no doubt full of oxytocin. We didn't return to our former "good" relationship because that one had been weaker and less mature. Our new bond more completely characterized the idea of being one flesh, taking us into a healthier future.

What about those situations that wound us but for which no reconciliation seems possible? Are we meant to fool ourselves into feeling no pain? Distract ourselves with happy thoughts? No. Our identity must be able to withstand the rigors of real life. Authenticity is a trait of regeneration. When we are fashioned into our best true self, we can face the truth about our situations without being destroyed by them.

This living into our true self is perhaps the longest phase in our transformative healing. It is so tempting to wish others would change—or even more, that we would change into a personality more pleasing than the one we have. But all the practices of those fruits of the Spirit don't change our uniqueness. We are made for unity in diversity, not identical identities. In this reality, there is always a tension back and forth, always feedback loops both biochemically and socially as we adjust to each other's claims on our lives. The Christ in us is surely all loving, but the expression of that Christ is deeply intertwined with the expressions of our true self.

Just as the body has spontaneous connections that are made in response to signals sent when wounds need healing, so our corporate body will need to make space for spontaneous connections to shape our healing pathways. Opening ourselves to interruptions on behalf of others, offering hospitality to someone who annoys us, and building enough margin into our days to notice and attend to the struggles within and outside ourselves make the powerful currents of transformation possible. The concepts of kinship in the body of Christ, hope, identity in the Trinity, and imagination are essential to transformative healing. Calling on the power of nonlocal healing through the eternal processes of prayer and loving relationships will always be inexplicable but real "alternative and complementary" factors in healing for people of faith. Much will remain a mystery, but the healing power of love has a brilliant clarity.

HISTORIES AND POTENTIALS

Wholeness and Healing in the Body

Our wounds become wombs.

ATTRIBUTED TO JULIAN OF NORWICH

UNTOUCHABLES. That word has special meaning in some cultures. When I worked in India, I met many members of the lowest caste, the Dalits, who are known by this term. Those with leprosy also became members of the Untouchables. When these patients came into the hospital, they expected me to draw back from physically examining them. Reflexively, they took off their sandals and showed me their lesions so I wouldn't have to touch them and thereby debase myself. Signs in the Christian hospital discouraged this kind of exclusionary thinking and instead encouraged patients to receive health care to free them from oppression: "Leprosy is the chief source of beggary" read one. Restored health was promoted as a way out of caste suffering.

Of course, I did touch the patients. Perhaps they chalked that up to my foreign ignorance more than to my faith. But I have treated untouchables in the United States, too. Forever etched in my memory is Belinda, a migrant farmworker in North Carolina. She'd been traded up and down the East Coast from farm to farm and from man to man. When I saw her in the clinic, she was downcast, a word evocative of the Dalit.

Haltingly, she told me there wasn't much I could do. She was just tired and needed something to help her rest. Her lungs ached and her night sweats wore her out. Belinda had AIDS, diagnosed in the days when we were just beginning to understand the heterosexual spread of the disease in primary care. She instinctively leaned away from me when she talked, sitting with slumped shoulders and speaking in a muffled voice.

Perhaps just as instinctively, when Belinda stood to leave, I gave her a hug. She froze. Then she cried and met my eyes. No one, she told me, touched her anymore. She hadn't been hugged in such a long time. It was what I could do.

All societies, including our own, have their untouchables. People who are beyond our circle of concern. People somehow not related to us, not deserving of our time and attention, and certainly not worth the risking of our own health for theirs. Even religions support these ideas—from ancient Judaism to present-day Hinduism, we see spiritual justifications for consigning some to lives of suffering.

But Jesus radically upended this sort of thinking. He touched those with leprosy, he healed the bleeding woman, and he spat on the blind man's eyes. He allowed himself to become unclean in the process of restoring health to those who seemed spiritually, as well as physically, beyond care. In speaking to the paralytic, he admonished that all healing, whether bodily or relationally, is a gift from God.[1] And when he shared his body and blood at the Last Supper, and later on the cross, he established a new connection, both mystical and corporate, between all who follow him.[2]

The early church understood the countercultural expression of sacrificially caring for those in need of healing. The hospitality shown to those with disabilities, ailments, and stigmatic diseases is thought to have been a significant factor in the early growth of the church.[3] In the fourth century, St. Basil the Great established the first hospital for the poor, welcoming those who had been driven out of cities because of their diseases.[4] The monks attending the sick knew they were at risk for becoming ill. Though they often had little to offer but comfort and companionship, they saw this work as vital to understanding how the body of Christ is displayed in the world.

Perhaps most people continue to associate Christianity with a concern for physical health and healing, rooted in our belief in the sanctity of life, as well as the dignity and image of God present in all humans. There are still many missional efforts in medicine. But for the most part, we leave physical healing to the professionals. In affluent parts of the world, we take most of our physical healing for granted, calling on God only when we are worried about something serious.

For a faith made distinct by the Incarnation and Resurrection, the centrality of the body seems an essential tenet. Yet so often we behave like disconnected beings, thinking and speaking on matters of faith but not grounding our day-to-day experiences in the fleshing out of those words we claim to believe. Attending to healing, in every aspect of our gathered lives, is and will always be a Christian vocation. It is not just for those with special gifts, but a call that encompasses us all. Comforting those who hurt, feeding the hungry, visiting the lonely, and extending hospitality to those whose views counter our own illustrate our vital connections to the body of Christ.

This book is an attempt to reclaim a unitive understanding of healing as a Christian ideal. Jesus showed first-century Hebrews that their expectations about the power of God's love were too narrow, too low. His message is still needed in our fractured and fragmented world. How is it that we so readily give up on a healing that may yet be possible, if only we have faith to see?

Our bodies are made to heal. We have built-in mechanisms that respond to wounds. As humans, we somehow recognize that we will be hurt and that woundedness is part of what it means to be alive. But because of the amazing design of our bodies, our injuries don't have to have the last word. Repair, restoration, and even regeneration bear witness to the possibility of full healing from our wounds.

Many question the relevance of the church today. Perhaps knowing the power of the body of Christ to stop the bleeding

and restore broken relationships, to clear away viral preju-
dices and misunderstandings, to give new shape to distorted
identities, and to collectively participate in the healing of
our untouchable places would draw people into the church,
much like the ancient ministries of physical healing did for
earlier cultures. It is still countercultural to include outcasts
and to create spaces where all are not only welcome, but also
viewed as vital to the life of the whole community.

Clotting, inflammation, tissue building, and remodeling—
these are our images for wound healing. Urgency and perseverance both have their place, as do personal transformation
and visionary hope. Despite our desires for expediency, we
aren't given a set of directions for assembling a conflict-free
life. Tension, pain, and death all play roles in the story of
healing from our wounds.

Our healing is full of paradox, which is again an image of
the Christian life. We follow a Savior who lived a perfect life
only to die as a criminal. Our God is one and three, our body
is one and many, and it is in dying that we have eternal life.
As we face the reality of our deeply wounded places, we have
the opportunity to more fully participate in being people
of regeneration. As Richard Rohr reflects, "Being wounded
and surviving helps us understand the pattern of life-death-
resurrection. We are no longer simply victims but empow-
ered and wise healers. No wonder the image of the Risen
Christ is still wounded."[5]

The apostle Paul writes that we are meant to "complete
what is lacking" in Christ's suffering (Colossians 1:24). That

seems strange and almost heretical. Didn't Christ's agonizing death complete the breach between humans and God, once and for all? But this passage is found in the context of a longer message that emphasizes Christ is the head of his body, which is the church. Paul recognizes that as we are joined to Christ's body, we are joined into his suffering—a suffering that is always on behalf of others. Eugene Peterson paraphrases these verses: "There's a lot of suffering to be entered into in this world—the kind of suffering Christ takes on. I welcome the chance to take my share in the church's part of that suffering."[6]

Suffering is something we so want to avoid. But it isn't the last word. It is just a way through. The body, both physically and mystically, is made for healing. What would our communities and congregations look like if we lived wholeheartedly into this truth? May our wounds become wombs.

ACKNOWLEDGMENTS

Jennie

As a reader, I typically glance over acknowledgments to learn a bit more about who matters to the author. It has always made sense to me to honor family members, those who reviewed early manuscripts, and anyone who contributed to research. But I never understood the heartfelt gratitude often directed to the editors and publisher.

Now I do.

From acquisition to manuscript completion, the editors and team at Tyndale House Publishers have been wonderful partners in this work. Jon Farrar and Kim Miller believed in this book's message and made it clearer and crisper with their input. They challenged me to share more of my own story than I might have and helped me see areas that I had missed or that needed to be better developed. Editing may conjure up a severe cutting of favorite phrases, but in reality, editing adds more than it takes away. To top it off, the editors are fun people! I'm so glad for my new relationships with Tyndale and so grateful they took a chance with Bem and me.

Philip Yancey gave us the incredible gift of his time, perspective, and experience. We received that with wonder and still hold his generous encouragement as a cherished treasure. His frank and kind critique shaped the book as well as our experience of being new authors.

Our champion is Luci Shaw. She pestered me into perseverance. She read every word of every draft, offered suggestions graciously and shared her excitement abundantly as she helped us visualize a completed manuscript.

Greg Johnson, our agent at WordServe Literary, enthusiastically welcomed us and guided us expertly in the process of securing a publisher. His integrity and sense of vocation undergird all he does.

The friends and family section could be unwieldy as Bem and I are blessed with numerous members across multiple continents. We are thankful for the ability to research and write while loved ones cared for daily needs. We are grateful for all the prayers and positivity we've received along the way. A special shout-out to my soul sisters, who embraced this book concept on our retreat.

My daughter Maggie read early drafts, cheered me on, and helped me try to reach an audience that isn't narrowly defined by one spiritual or social viewpoint.

And Andrew—how can I truly acknowledge his role in all this? He always treats my writing as a valid enterprise, regardless of its ultimate use. His sacrifices give me the time and space to follow a line of words. He knows how many times

I have been the wounder as well as the wounded, and yet he promotes restoration, renewal, and hope time and again.

Bem is knit forever into the tissue of my life. What a joy.

Bem

I am so grateful to Jennie for bringing me into the ministry of harmonizing the divided worlds of science and faith, as well as welcoming me into her remarkable family and circle of friends. Jennie's talent, determination, sacrifice, and courage to write this book inspired me throughout our miraculous journey.

Julio, my husband, took a huge risk in marrying a badly wounded and scarred woman. His patient love has brought great healing and joy to my life. Our partnership and his gourmet cooking have sustained me during my scientific career and the long nights spent working on this book. I offered our son, Caleb, the power of censorship over our personal stories so he wouldn't be inadvertently publicly embarrassed or hurt. He reviewed my drafts and relinquished the gift: "Mom, it's your story. Tell it the way you want to." His maturity, humor, and brilliant jazz guitar playing got us through many difficult conversations about his and his generation's outlook on the subject matter.

Biologist Kristie Fox and engineer Jed Brewer reviewed the science narratives and helped me provide feedback to Jennie. Robin and Roger Stoller modeled the healing power of community and helped my family survive many crises, enabling me to work during these tumultuous times. My knowledge on tissue healing is largely due to research supported by these business partners and collaborators: Tracy Warren, Joe Oswald, Mila and Jerry Tate, Bill Malkes, and the Stollers. Their belief that faith enriches science and vice versa gave me complete freedom to coauthor this book while keeping my day job.

REFLECTION AND DISCUSSION GUIDE

For Individual Readers or Small Groups

BY ENTERING ONE FAMILY'S STORY, you can navigate the possible responses that may develop as a wound is experienced over time. Clotting, inflammation, tissue formation, scarring, and restoration will promote healing, while overactive reactions, proud flesh, lack of closure, and binding contractures will threaten resolution.

As you consider the images introduced in each chapter, we encourage you to ponder your own experiences and how you tend to respond to such events. There are a variety of possible reactions to each situation; hopefully, you and/or your discussion group will make the simple fictional story a robust platform for engaging in reflection or discussion about injuries that fester in your own life or local contexts.

CHAPTER 1

Martin and Andrea Cruz are married with three young children, ages fifteen months to seven years. Martin is employed in the construction industry, and Andrea works for the federal government. Her job often requires travel, and they've moved three times in the past five years due to her promotions.

Over the past two years, Andrea's father's health has deteriorated due to a fairly rapid onset of dementia. She and Martin struggle in their response to this situation, disagreeing on the best way to support her parents. They also feel pressure from her older brother and sister to be supportive and present in ways that disrupt their own family life. Andrea, the youngest of the three siblings, is the only one who has moved far from their hometown.

As Christmas approaches, the issues come to a head. Andrea has been traveling most of the autumn, and she feels fatigued. Martin wants to stay home and relax with their children and close friends. The baby still isn't sleeping through the night, which would make staying in a hotel or with relatives difficult. However, Andrea's two siblings tell her that this Christmas might be the last one her father can really participate in and insist that it is essential that she and the children celebrate the holiday with her parents and siblings.

For Andrea and Martin, traveling back to her hometown would mean spending money on airline fares at peak prices. After suggesting they come in the new year instead, the couple is met with a fiery barrage of emails from Andrea's siblings, who express outrage at the insensitivity she and Martin are showing to their mother and father. Andrea seems able to travel for work; why can't she travel for family? She moved far from the family's home and doesn't help out on a weekly basis like the others do. They also insinuate that Martin is contributing to the rupture of the tight family bonds the siblings once enjoyed. In truth, Martin, whose family has been estranged since his parents' divorce, doesn't understand the guilt and sadness Andrea expresses at the thought of not visiting her parents and siblings this Christmas.

Questions for Reflection and Discussion

1. Who do you most identify with in this story?

2. What wounds do you notice in this family? Which one needs the most urgent attention now?

3. If you were to play the role of the individual with whom you most closely identify, what do you think you should do now to promote healing?

4. How do you find yourself responding to this story? Is it familiar? Fear-provoking or painful? Have you seen families successfully negotiate this sort of wound without it becoming chronic or extreme? What characterized any healthy responses you have witnessed?

CHAPTER 2

It's almost December, and Andrea's family are still after her to come home for Christmas. Her siblings have sent her proposed itineraries that could save money on travel and have offered to pick up the family from the airport. Seeing the toll this is taking on his wife, Martin suggests they block their phones from the siblings for a while, or at least ignore their advice. Andrea disagrees, as she fears being cut off from important news about her dad. She is torn, thinking perhaps it would be best just to go there for Christmas.

One Saturday, Andrea proposes to Martin that she take the baby so the two of them can spend Christmas with her parents and siblings. It would just be this once, and the baby would fly free. Martin explodes, "Are you kidding? Break up *our* family so *your* family can be satisfied? They're never satisfied! What's next? Moving back there?" Left unacknowledged—even to himself—is the resentment he feels as the parent who always has to pick up the slack at home. More than that, he is beginning to feel neglected by Andrea, whose energy all seems to be directed at her job, the children, and her parents.

Andrea begins sobbing. Her style is to retreat when hurt. She cries, "I'm trapped! I can't win! No matter what, Christmas will be sad. Our children don't deserve this stress, and neither do I! I'm going out to clear my head."

As she slams the front door behind her, Andrea is numb and confused. She calls her friend Teresa, whom she met through the book group Teresa leads, asking if she can come by. Teresa is quite a bit older than Andrea and emigrated from Vietnam shortly after her marriage. She has often shared how difficult it was for her to juggle all her responsibilities without family nearby.

Questions for Reflection and Discussion

1. What current wound in the Cruz family needs urgent attention?

2. A healthy defense requires prompt action, clot formation to stop the bleeding, positive pressure to control the damage, and a clearing of debris. What would that look like in this situation?

3. What role might Teresa play? Consider responses you would want Teresa to give as well as responses you would want her to avoid. What roles could Andrea and Martin play in clot formation right now?

4. There has been no mention of a discernment process for Martin and Andrea. We don't know how they are trying to understand their own roles apart from just reacting to the energy of the moment. The concerns shared so far have all been pragmatic or emotional. What are some practices that could help them both move to a calmer space as they consider the best way forward? What practices do they need to avoid? Who else could they call upon to help them resolve their wound?

5. How, if at all, should they engage with Andrea's family right now? How might Andrea's mom or her siblings bring positive pressure to the situation? Is there a way any one of them might clear debris?

CHAPTER 3

Sitting in Teresa's kitchen, Andrea spills out her confusion, anger, and sadness while Teresa comforts her with tea, sweets, and a soothing presence. While Andrea doesn't leave with a specific plan, she returns home with a desire to heal this latest fiery episode with Martin. It seems as if Martin has some sort of outburst whenever they bring up her family's situation. Andrea wants these episodes to end.

Despite her good intentions, Andrea realizes she needs to start supper for the children as soon as she gets home. After that, they need baths, and then Andrea has to respond to several work emails.

Over the next week, Andrea has little time to sit down and discuss the situation with Martin. Whenever she proposes that they find a time to talk through the issue, she is met with comments like these:

"Not now, when I finally get a chance to relax after a long day."

"You know, we have bills to pay, and you agreed we'd talk about our budget."

"I don't see the point in talking; your family always gets their way. Do what you want!"

As the days go by, the tension between them grows. One day as Martin fixes lunch for the children, Andrea begins packing for her last work trip of the year. The little ones are in the family room watching a video when she hears the distinctive ringtone on Martin's phone.

"Hey, Bill," Andrea hears him say. She sighs. Martin

is rarely in a good mood after talking with his supervisor. "I can't go to that site until Monday afternoon because my wife is heading out of town." After a moment of silence, he adds, "I know, I'm not happy about it either. Yes, I can try to figure out something with my kids." A few seconds later, she hears Martin mutter, "See ya, Bill." Then she hears him kick the wastebasket.

Martin comes into the bedroom and tells Andrea she has to figure out a different day-care arrangement because he needs to be able to do his job. "Instead of figuring out how to be with your family, why don't you figure out how to be with *this* family!" After a brief pause, he adds, "And by the way—just because you make twice as much as I do doesn't mean all the childcare should fall on me."

Andrea silently picks up her suitcase and heads for the door.

Questions for Reflection and Discussion

1. What is happening to the original wound between Andrea's family of origin and her current nuclear family? What is disordered in the current inflammatory process?

2. Martin seems to be the one making things worse here. But how might his history—his parents' divorce; concern over his boss's displeasure at his inability to visit job sites whenever Andrea travels; lack of free time or time with friends—contribute to chronic inflammation?

3. Andrea wants to smooth things over. When we
    consider the image of an ulcer, what does smoothing it
    over accomplish? How might she and Martin address
    the chronic inflammation without making it flare up,
    fester, or get more deeply under their skin?

4. Imagine that you are a mediator preparing to sit down
    with Martin and Andrea. What do you think they need
    to do to prepare to discuss their family issues? What
    needs to be out in the open? How might you counsel
    them regarding managing their expectations? How
    might gratitude play a role in this scenario?

5. As they were growing up, Martin and Andrea had very
    different experiences of a nuclear family. Consider how
    they might allow those past histories to be constructive,
    rather than destructive, in reducing inflammation
    now. How might stigma be a part of this inflammatory
    response? How might they address that?

6. What does this chapter on disordered inflammation
    conjure up for you? Does the term *culture of outrage*
    ring true? Consider how it might be helpfully addressed
    at your workplace or school, or in your neighborhood
    or faith community.

CHAPTER 4

Pressure is building in the Cruz marriage. Meanwhile, Andrea's
siblings are experiencing their own increasing stress. Carmen,

Andrea's sister, has been researching treatment protocols for dementia and is trying to get her parents to agree to her father's participation in a clinical trial offered in a university medical center about seventy miles from their home. Her parents are reluctant to leave the care of their longtime family doctor.

Thomas, Andrea's brother, is preoccupied with his concerns about his parents' safety in their family home and is urging them to move into a senior care center. That idea also meets strong resistance from his parents. With each day that passes, Thomas feels growing dread over his parents' declining health.

Carmen is a homemaker and often feels she is unfairly relied upon to respond to last-minute requests from her parents to help with errands, appointment scheduling, and household needs. She has little personal time.

One day Carmen tells Andrea about another complication over the phone. She explains that their mom called that morning. In a shaky voice, she told Carmen, "Your father and I have been in a car wreck! Don't get upset. We're okay, but the car needs towing. The airbags went off."

Carmen immediately asked her mom what happened and where they were. She learned that their mother didn't stop quickly enough approaching an intersection and rear-ended the car in front of her. No one was hurt, but their mom was cited for being at fault.

Carmen rushed to the scene. She tells Andrea that their father was clearly confused about the day's circumstances. They'd been on their way to a doctor's appointment.

"I normally drive them places," Carmen said, choking up, "but I told them I was busy this morning. And Andrea, Thomas blew up when he learned about the accident. He said, 'I told you, Carmen, that if you can't drive them someplace, they need a driver! They need to get out of that house before one of them kills the other through incompetence! We need to make them move!'" Andrea tries to comfort her sister, even as guilt and worry flood through her, too.

After a flurry of phone calls, the family members agree to an urgent family meeting. Andrea and Martin will join by conference call. Their aunt Ruth, their mother's younger sister, volunteers to stay at the family home for the next week, wanting to be helpful as a driver and calm presence. She is known for her listening ear, loud laughter, and abundant dinners.

Aunt Ruth's presence on the call does cut through some of the tension. After acknowledging the pressures on and contributions of each person, she asks questions and listens. As her nieces and nephew struggle to determine next steps, Aunt Ruth suggests using a faith-based elder-care network. This ministry provides print, video, and in-person discussion resources on how to navigate the best course for aging family members. Two families at Ruth's church have used this group with great results, and they've offered to speak with Ruth's extended family.

Ruth suggests they all gather in person after the holidays at a comfortable lodge near her home where they can all be on neutral ground. There are lots of fun kids' activities there, and January prices make it affordable. They won't have to worry about meals either.

Andrea breathes a sigh of relief when Thomas says, "That sounds like a great idea!" and Carmen agrees. Suddenly she knows her immediate family has found a way out of the earlier Christmas dilemma. Rather than go during the holiday, they can fly to Andrea's hometown for a shorter stay in January, when airline tickets will be less expensive.

Right after Christmas, Aunt Ruth sends a proposed schedule for their family retreat and welcomes everyone to suggest modifications. Included is an afternoon meeting with several seniors and caregivers from the elder-care network who will share their stories and relate both the good and bad aspects of their various decisions. A leader in the network will facilitate, and Aunt Ruth tells her family that this person has invited each family member (and spouse) to confidentially email her with their questions, concerns, fears, hopes, resources, and constraints related to elder care within their family.

Questions for Reflection and Discussion

1. As we think about the risk of compartment syndrome, what compartments or family bundles do you recognize? How does one affect the pressure in the other? How do we navigate relieving such widespread tension when people are hurting within their own compressed spaces? Do you have examples of this in your life? If so, which one comes to mind first?

2. If this family's well-being is to be preserved, these high pressures need to be relieved by a flaying open, exposing all the wounded spots so regeneration can occur. Who might help with that? Do you have examples from your own life of a skilled "surgeon" in the context of conflict?

3. We know some of the issues that are important to the siblings. What about the parents' desires? How might they be best addressed?

4. How might the elder-care network suggested by Aunt Ruth reflect ideas discussed as part of the Table of Significant Others (TOSO) tool (see pages 100–101)? What types of people may need to speak into this situation for it to resolve well?

5. How is Aunt Ruth like fibronectin? What do you think should happen between now and January to assist holding the tension in life-giving ways? Who has been like fibronectin in your life? How can you be more like that in a place that needs healing?

6. How might Aunt Ruth's agenda help give personal voice and agency to all the siblings? What about the parents? The spouses? Does this scenario seem realistic, or too complex to be possible? In your own life, are there pieces of such a gathering that you can envision to address multilayered conflict?

7. The issue of grief and death has not been given voice. Yet it is the constant undercurrent as siblings worry about a "last Christmas," Thomas fears his parents' impending incompetence, and their mother wants to hang on to her house and the physician they've grown to trust. How often do grief and the reality of death remain hidden in situations of family conflict? What are some healthy ways to mediate this problem?

CHAPTER 5

Andrea's extended family manages to make it through the holidays without another crisis. Martin and Andrea choose to mark their own Christmas with some new traditions, taking their family caroling and attending a candlelight service geared toward children. Feeling buoyed by the relative calm, everyone comes to the January retreat with hopeful expectations of unity. The cousins have a great time swimming in the indoor water park and playing mini golf. Andrea's parents dote on her children, and Aunt Ruth supplies everyone with her tastiest baked goods.

Andrea's mother has told her that she's made a decision to quit driving, so that issue is resolved. Her parents are firm in their decision not to pursue the experimental treatment for her father. However, now it is more important than ever to determine whether the family home should be sold. As the adults gather for their sessions with the elder-care network representatives, it is clear to all that independent living is no longer a healthy option for their parents. Andrea and her siblings gather information on a number of adult care homes in the area, including the financial costs. Wanting to verify the decision in front of everyone, Thomas asks his parents if they are willing to sell their house and move by early summer, and his parents say they are.

The rest of the time together goes well, as everyone is at ease with the choices they've made. Andrea's siblings agree to monthly check-ins to discuss progress and needs. Thomas will fix up the house to sell, and Carmen plans to sort through their parents' belongings. Andrea takes responsibility for investigating legal issues such as power of attorney and estate planning. A few weeks after the retreat, she calls her mother to verify that her parents have a will and gather the additional information she will need for the attorney.

Her mother's comments throw her. "Honey, we have a will, but I'm going to change it. I really don't want to go to an assisted living place. I talked to Carmen and asked her if we could turn over the proceeds from the sale of our house to her so they can build an addition on their home for Daddy and me. We will still have money for in-home care if we need it. I think Daddy will go downhill fast if we move to some place with old folks."

Andrea's thoughts race. *Does Thomas know about this? Is Carmen happy about it? Now Carmen will get all the equity in the sale of the house. How is that fair?* Is Andrea just out of sight, out of mind? She is always the last to know, and her opinion doesn't seem to matter anyway. As soon as Andrea hangs up with her mom, she calls Carmen.

"How could you go behind my back and change everything we agreed on?" she asks. "You always say you need help, and now you are going to have them live with you? You must be planning a fancy addition! All of Mom and Daddy's money will be sunk into your house! How do you expect me to help with estate planning when you are taking their estate!"

Carmen says very little during Andrea's outburst. Then she tells Andrea that it was their mother's idea and that Thomas thinks it is okay. Carmen says she thought it through and believes that with in-home help, the plan could work for everyone. She and Thomas assumed Andrea and Martin would be fine with the change since it doesn't require any extra effort on their part. Plus, they already have secure financial investments. Carmen and her husband could help her parents now and have better financial security in the future.

Andrea calls Thomas next. He says he doesn't see any issues with the revised plan. He would rather have the situation handled than worry about the finances that might be left after their parents die. In any event, their mom told Thomas she is giving Thomas her car since she no longer needs it.

"How convenient," Andrea mutters.

"Hey!" Thomas said. "You do realize I'm the backup driver for Mom and Dad, right?"

Questions for Reflection and Discussion

1. Andrea assumes the family's healing is progressing nicely, and then she is thrown for a loop. What do you think? Is her anger justified? How might you take the side of each family member here?

2. Proud flesh happens after a good initial start to healing. It is lopsided growth outside the boundary lines of the wound space. How do the issues of the will and the home addition expand the boundary lines of the original wound? How are they affecting the original complaint?

3. Even if others' actions cause hurt, proud flesh develops when we attempt to control the response of those who we perceive may harm us. How could Andrea reimagine her boundary lines as pleasant, her "inheritance" as good? What does she need to relinquish for that to happen?

4. Has proud flesh developed in any of your areas of conflict? Chronic friction causes proud flesh. How might chronic friction—whether about how you perceive you are valued or the ways that communication breaks down—be addressed regularly as soon as you sense it disrupting an almost-healed space? Recall how the church planter abstained from complaint (see pages 113–114). Is there such a practice you could undertake or consider?

5. Why is rewounding necessary to eliminate proud flesh in this scenario? How might Andrea, Carmen, and Thomas broach this new hurt—Andrea feeling sidelined—in a safe way that will allow them to move forward?

CHAPTER 6

Andrea is still livid over the planned expansion to Carmen's home when she arrives home that evening. To her surprise, Martin doesn't react to the situation as strongly as she did. He reminds her that a financial inheritance is always an elusive good that cannot be counted upon. Ideally, it is a gift, not a demand. They aren't depending on anything from her parents, and her mother may live many more years anyway. This new plan will help resolve the needs of her parents, so why not just agree to it?

Through discussions with Martin, her friend Teresa, and her aunt Ruth, Andrea realizes it really isn't even about the money. It is about her sense of place in the family, her status as a beloved child. She writes her mother an honest letter about feeling left out, and her mom responds with apologies and kind affirmations. She tells Andrea she was just trying to be practical, not to demonstrate love for one child over another.

Several months later, the calls between the siblings resume. Andrea asks that they share any significant decisions they make with her right away to prevent hurtful surprises.

Her siblings agree. Thomas says he doesn't understand why Andrea had been so upset in the first place, but he'll go along with her request. Carmen suggests that if anyone has questions or concerns about future financial decisions, they agree to resolve them before moving on. Carmen notes that the financial piece can be a burden as well as a benefit; undertaking daily care for their parents is complex. Then she asks if Andrea would like to be in charge of the upcoming estate sale they will hold after the sale of the house.

The family plans one last gathering in their parents' home. They reminisce about the holidays they've shared, laugh at the penciled marks on the basement wall documenting their growth over the years, and marvel at how tall the trees they helped plant many years ago have become. Carmen surprises everyone with their own photo album, which chronicles their years in the house.

Questions for Reflection and Discussion

1. By the time Carmen, Thomas, and Andrea make a final visit to their childhood home, it seems the family's major initial wounds have finally reached closure. How does the story reflect aspects of scar formation?

2. While in treatment for some of his own wounds, pastor and author Mike Erre said he was told, "You can share scars, but don't share wounds" (see page 131). Andrea shares her wound with her mother but not her siblings. How do you react to this idea of wounds versus scars,

and to how Andrea deals with her hurt? How do we discern whom to reveal our scars to? Our fresh wounds?

3. The siblings understand the importance of Andrea's wound differently. Is this typical in your experience? Why and when does it matter?

4. Scars tell stories, acting as maps of memory. How is this new scar formation in Andrea's family allowing all their past wounds and reconciliation attempts to be gathered into fibrin strands that weave together to provide closure?

5. Our scars can act as an Ebenezer—a reminder of God's help in the past and our hope for the future. In Andrea's case, the photo album Carmen has created and the final visit to the family home may serve as an Ebenezer. In what situations have you placed an Ebenezer? Are there current scarring places you'd like to mark as hopeful signposts indicating a milestone in your journey toward healing?

6. What scars related to personal, community, religious, and/or national wounds would you like to see form and be recognized? How might you assist with that?

7. Scarring takes patience. How do you feel about the progress Andrea's extended family is making? Does it seem realistic to you? Why or why not? What might still threaten the tensile strength of the family's scar?

CHAPTER 7

Months later, the house has been sold, the addition built onto Carmen's home, and Andrea's parents are settled. The transition has gone smoothly overall, but there have been a few bumps along the way. Home health aides have been hard to find and retain. Their mother refuses to use a driver from Uber or other ride-sharing companies; instead, she wants Thomas to take over the driving since she gave him the car. Both parents have an increasing number of medical appointments, and Andrea's father is no longer able to be left safely by himself.

Andrea has finalized the estate sale and is the legally appointed financial guardian for her parents. One day her mother calls, saying she wants to "discuss some loose ends that need to be tied up."

"Sweetie," her mom asks, "what needs to happen so Thomas can be in charge of the finances now that you have made things so organized?"

Andrea is stunned. She has done such a good job with her parents' finances, and yet her mother wants her to hand over all her work!

"Mom! You're doing it again! You're devaluing me! Thomas isn't as good with money as I am. He doesn't even care about details. Why are you suggesting a change now?"

"I just think it's more practical, honey, since you live so far away," her mom says. "Thomas could go to the bank to get me cash or something from our safety deposit box when I need it." She adds that she plans to make a few additional changes to her will and wants some financial advice for that.

She thinks working with a local financial adviser, assisted by Thomas, would be best.

Andrea immediately feels anger toward Thomas rising up in her. As if her mother senses that, she says, "I mentioned this to Thomas, and he said I should talk to you about it and see what you think. I asked Carmen to take over the finances first, but she said she already has too much to do."

Questions for Reflection and Discussion

1. Andrea's scars seem to be pretty itchy. Hypersensitivity is setting in, with puffy overgrowth. What is your response to this turn of events? What is contributing to scar adhesion and contracture?

2. What do you think should happen now? How can the family stop and trace their scar's journey? Is there any stigma at this point that is affecting growth?

3. Where might Andrea and her family find healthy community? Imagine what sort of community might assist them. How might community embrace this family and tug on the scar in such a way that it doesn't break open?

4. What words or actions would you advise Andrea or other family members to avoid? In what ways have your scars been affected by keloid or hypertrophy? What helped you resolve that distorted remodeling of what had been a closed, past wound?

CHAPTER 8

A year after her parents' move, Andrea and Martin are both in stable jobs. They have joined a church that is quite active in their city, and now that Andrea's parents are well cared for, they are considering how to participate in it more fully. One of the congregation's leaders recently moved from Chicago, where she was engaged with a movement called Renew Chicago (renewChicago.city). The Cruzes' church decides to initiate a similar work in their own town. They see it as a transformational opportunity, a new creation to overcome a legacy of racism and oppression that is countercultural to the gospel message.

The work of renewal is open to anyone in their community who is interested. All faith communities in the area are invited to take part, though it clearly operates from a Christian worldview. Like the work in Chicago, they hope to develop concrete programs of renewal in schools, neighborhoods, economic development, and leadership.

Andrea and Martin both contribute to the work, finding it brings joy and a new dimension to their family life. Andrea, known for her national work in intercultural dialogue, is invited to be on the founding board. She is gratified to see her ideas being valued and taken seriously, and Martin is able to put his construction skills to use as the church renovates an abandoned storefront to serve as a tutoring center and food pantry. Whenever someone compliments one spouse on the work he or she is doing, the other beams with pride.

Questions for Reflection and Discussion

1. How has the healing of Andrea's family wound created space for her and Martin to pursue new interests and work to help transform lives in their own community? What lessons and interpersonal skills from the earlier situation may be valuable as they join in this new work?

2. Scarless healing happens best in the fetus, as the body is being formed. In other words, it is not a response to old wounds but to birth defects. Visit Renew Chicago's website (renewChicago.city). How is it an example of a new birth? Can we expect any kind of scarless healing when dealing with legacies of injustice?

3. What do you think Scripture has to say about our hopes for transformation on earth? Some theologies hold to transforming culture, some to standing against culture, and others to a paradox of doing all we can while knowing it will not be enough. How do you engage in hopeful work in our culture if you are a Christian? If you aren't a Christian, what is your "theology of culture"?

4. As you consider this church-based renewal work, what features do you see that would promote rapid healing? What should be included as growth factors, mediators, fibronectin, and the tug of healthy community?

5. Bem's mice did just fine until they were born. What will be needed to sustain the work of projects like

Renew Chicago after they are birthed? How will the Cruzes' city learn to operate as a mature environment, or will it always need a renewal program such as this one?

6. Where do you long for scarless healing? Where do you believe it is not realistic and maybe even harmful?

CHAPTER 9

"In social healing, deep transformation of relationships must take place. We change our minds about each other and ourselves" (page 192).

As Andrea and Martin join others in working for renewal within the city, they must discern what new opportunities they are called to be part of in a healing transformation that extends far beyond their families of origin. New models of cooperative housing are being planned, and the Cruz family is considering a move into the heart of the city.

However, because the couple can't be sure of the outcome of such an effort, they are weighing the potential benefits and costs. It seems like a significant way to participate in inclusive transformation, but will their children be safe, have friends, and get a decent education? How long will it take for the generational stresses in the community to be reduced—will it even be possible in their lifetimes? There is so much need everywhere they look. They are torn as they try to understand their own role in this time and place.

Questions for Reflection and Discussion

1. Have you been drawn to a work that is focused on transformation of a system or social structure that has borne a legacy of stress and wounding? What do you notice in that situation that resonates with the relationship between chronic stress and resulting social discord?

2. If you were able to talk with Andrea and Martin about their situation, what questions would you ask? What advice would you offer from your own viewpoint and experience? How do we balance the claims upon us to work for the healing of the world while attending to our own health and that of our family?

3. Where have you seen the interplay of mind, body, and spirit in healing either physical or social wounds?

4. Have you experienced a placebo effect? Does the information in the chapter make you rethink any skepticism you may have about how people respond to various interventions directed at their healing?

5. How do you respond to the idea of practicing a behavior until it forms "grooves" (page 200) and takes root in a meaningful way?

6. When you think of your identity, what words come to mind? Racial and gender identity occupy much of our

current public discourse. How do these two aspects shape your own identity? Do you experience a kinship with those whose racial, gender, cultural, religious, and social identities are different from yours? If so, how has that come to be?

7. What core identity do you long for? What keeps that from fully shaping your life?

CHAPTER 10

As we close this book discussion, review the chapters and consider what aspects of healing most significantly speak to you at this moment of your life:

Clotting, inflammation, tissue building, and remodeling—these are our images for wound healing. Urgency and perseverance both have their place, as do personal transformation and visionary hope. Despite our desires for expediency, we aren't given a set of directions for assembling a conflict-free life. Tension, pain, and death all play roles in the story of healing from our wounds.

Designed to Heal, PAGE 209

Questions for Reflection and Discussion

1. Have you tried to model any of the practices described in the book? Which ones?

2. As you consider the stages of clotting, inflammation, tissue building, and remodeling, which do you see as the most difficult to engage? How might it be made more possible to attain?

3. What particular corporate wounds (in family, work relationships, society, faith communities, etc.) do you see as most urgent to address? Why? If healing has begun, in what stage of healing is this wound? Is it stuck in a particular stage or mending adequately?

4. How hopeful are you that the entrenched wounds you experience can be transformed? How might you give hope to others? What steps you want to take in being a part of a healing community?

NOTES

INTRODUCTION: BODIES

1. The stories of Elijah and other patients in this book are true, but names and identifying characteristics have been altered to protect their privacy.
2. Abraham Kuyper, *Wisdom and Wonder: Common Grace in Science and Art* (Grand Rapids, MI: Christian's Library Press, 2011), 39.

CHAPTER 1: WOUNDED

1. Chandan K. Sen et al., "Human Skin Wounds: A Major and Snowballing Threat to Public Health and the Economy," *Wound Repair and Regeneration* 17, no. 6 (November–December 2009), 763–71, https://doi.org/10.1111/j.1524-475X.2009.00543.x.
2. Samuel R. Nussbaum et al., "An Economic Evaluation of the Impact, Cost, and Medicare Policy Implications of Chronic Nonhealing Wounds," *Value in Health* 21, no. 1 (January 2018), 27–32, https://doi.org/10.1016/j.jval.2017.07.007.
3. Dan J. White Jr., "Can the Church Overcome Polarization?" *Relevant*, July 22, 2019, https://www.relevantmagazine.com/faith/can-the-church-overcome-polarization/. This article is an excerpt from White's book *Love over Fear: Facing Monsters, Befriending Enemies, and Healing Our Polarized World* (Chicago: Moody Publishers, 2019).
4. See 1 Corinthians 12:12.

CHAPTER 2: FRESHLY INJURED

1. See pray-as-you-go.org.
2. See Allison Aubrey, "Feeling Anxious? Here's a Quick Tool to Center Your Soul," NPR, February 4, 2020, https://www.npr.org/2020/02/03/802347757/a-conversation-with-tara-brach-mindfulness-tools-for-big-feelings.

3. The storm also went by the name Typhoon Haiyan. See "Tropical Cyclone Case Study: Typhoon Haiyan," BBC, https://www.bbc.co.uk/bitesize /guides/z9whg82/revision/4.
4. Enjoli Francis and Eric Noll, "13 Truckers Create 'Safety Net' on Highway to Save Man Planning to Jump: Police," ABC News, April 25, 2018, https://abcnews.go.com/US/13-trucks-create-safety-net-highway-save-man /story?id=54734147.

CHAPTER 3: INFLAMMATION GONE AWRY
1. Alia Wong, "When the Last Patient Dies," *Atlantic*, May 27, 2015, https:// www.theatlantic.com/health/archive/2015/05/when-the-last-patient-dies /394163/.
2. Wong, "When the Last Patient Dies."
3. Puja Mehta et al., "COVID-19: Consider Cytokine Storm Syndromes and Immunosuppression," *Lancet* 395, no. 10229, (March 16, 2020): 1033–34, https://doi.org/10.1016/S0140-6736(20)30628-0.
4. Vocabulary.com, s.v. "inflammation," accessed December 8, 2020, https:// www.vocabulary.com/dictionary/inflammation.
5. Terri Apter, "The Dangerous Pleasures of Outrage," *Psychology Today*, March 22,2018, https://www.psychologytoday.com/us/blog/domestic -intelligence/201803/the-dangerous-pleasures-outrage.
6. Barbara L. Fredrickson, *Positivity: Groundbreaking Research Reveals How to Embrace the Hidden Strength of Positive Emotions, Overcome Negativity, and Thrive* (New York: Crown Publishing, 2009).
7. Lee Rainie and Andrew Perrin, "Key Findings about Americans' Declining Trust in Government and Each Other," Pew Research Center, July 22, 2019, https://www.pewresearch.org/fact-tank/2019/07/22/key-findings -about-americans-declining-trust-in-government-and-each-other/.
8. See Deuteronomy 5:15; 1 Chronicles 16:12, 15; Isaiah 46:9; Lamentations 3:21-24.
9. Mike Bundrant, "Three Delusions That Lead to Chronic Arguing, High Stress and Early Death," iNLP Center, https://inlpcenter.org/chronic -arguing-stress-death.
10. "Family Estrangement Survey for Stand Alone," Ipsos MORI website, October 7, 2014, https://www.ipsos.com/ipsos-mori/en-uk/family -estrangement-survey-stand-alone.
11. Christine Ro, "The Truth about Family Estrangement," BBC, March 31, 2019, https://www.bbc.com/future/article/20190328-family-estrangement -causes.

12. Richard P. Conti, "Family Estrangement: Establishing a Prevalence Rate," *Journal of Psychology and Behavioral Science* 3, no. 2 (December 2015): 28–35, https://doi.org/10.15640/jpbs.v3n2a4.

13. Terri Apter, "The Persistent Pain of Family Estrangement," *Psychology Today*, December 22, 2015, https://www.psychologytoday.com/us/blog /domestic-intelligence/201512/the-persistent-pain-family-estrangement; Lucy Blake, Becca Bland, and Susan Golombok, *Hidden Voices: Family Estrangement in Adulthood*, a report on research conducted in 2015 by the University of Cambridge Centre for Family Research and Stand Alone, https://www.standalone.org.uk/wp-content/uploads/2015/12/Hidden Voices.FinalReport.pdf.

14. Apter, "Persistent Pain."

15. Frederick Buechner, *Wishful Thinking: A Theological ABC* (New York: Harper & Row, 1973), 2.

16. "Constant Arguing 'Increases Premature Death Risk,'" BBC News, May 9, 2014, https://www.bbc.com/news/health-27327325.

17. Fredrickson, *Positivity*, 73.

18. Karen A. Wientjes, "Mind-Body Techniques in Wound Healing," *Ostomy/ Wound Management* 48, no. 11 (November 2002): 62–67, PMID: 12426453.

19. David Isay, *Listening Is an Act of Love: A Celebration of American Life from the StoryCorps Project* (New York: Penguin Press, 2007).

20. Gretchen Grappone, "Overcoming Stigma," National Alliance on Mental Illness, October 15, 2018, https://www.nami.org/Blogs/NAMI-Blog /October-2018/Overcoming-Stigma?fbclid=IwAR0JkhJPu9IALoW0AB JzdF3u1pI6maPfW-UrxAYVMCX5-uwW2r0dTzLUqIE.

21. "Strangers: Part Two," *This Is Us*, season 4, episode 18.

CHAPTER 4: VITAL CONNECTIONS

1. Karin Jewel Stone, "An Evaluation of Recidivism Rates for Resolutions Northwest's Victim-Offender Mediation Program, abstract (master's thesis, Portland State University, 2000), https://doi.org/10.15760/etd.2288.

2. Anders Hallengren, "Nelson Mandela and the Rainbow of Culture," NobelPrize.org, September 11, 2001, https://www.nobelprize.org/prizes /peace/1993/mandela/article.

3. Patrick Alexander and Otis W. Pickett, "The Prison-to-College Pipeline Program: An Ethical, Education-Based Response to Mass Incarceration in Mississippi," *Journal of African American History* 103, no. 4 (Fall 2018): 702–16, https://doi.org/10.1086/699955.

4. Lois M. Davis et al., "Evaluating the Effectiveness of Correctional Education: A Meta-Analysis of Programs That Provide Education to Incarcerated Adults," Rand Corporation, 2013, https://doi.org/10.7249 /RR266.

5. Parker J. Palmer, *Healing the Heart of Democracy: The Courage of Create a Politics Worthy of the Human Spirit* (San Francisco: Jossey-Bass, 2011), 6.

6. Palmer, *Healing the Heart of Democracy*, back cover.

7. Palmer, *Healing the Heart of Democracy*.

8. Rabbi Jeremy Kalmanofsky, "Every Bone in Your Body," Ansche Chesed blog, January 8, 2019, https://www.anschechesed.org/every-bone-in -your-body/.

9. Mark 12:28-31.

10. Simone Campbell, "Religion and Politics," *Oneing* 5, no. 2 (2017): 57–59.

CHAPTER 5: PROUD FLESH

1. Dan J. Stein et al., "The Impact of the Truth and Reconciliation Commission on Psychological Distress and Forgiveness in South Africa," *Social Psychiatry and Psychiatric Epidemiology* 43 (June 2008): 462–68. https://doi.org/10.1007/s00127-008-0350-0.

2. See John 5:1-12.

3. Psalm 16:6, NIV.

4. Richard Rohr, "Healthy Boundaries," Center for Action and Contemplation, December 4, 2016, https://cac.org/healthy-boundaries-2016-12-04/.

5. Rohr, "Healthy Boundaries."

CHAPTER 6: SCARRING AND MATURATION

1. Peter Mead, "Share Scars Not Wounds," Biblical Preaching, December 13, 2016, https://biblicalpreaching.net/2016/12/13/share-scars-not-wounds/.

2. For more on the history of the Vietnam Veterans Memorial, see the website for the Vietnam Veterans Memorial Fund, https://www.vvmf.org /About-The-Wall/history-of-the-vietnam-veterans-memorial/.

3. See 1 Samuel 7:3-14.

CHAPTER 7: IMPAIRED SCARRING

1. Clement D. Marshall et al., "Cutaneous Scarring: Basic Science, Current Treatments, and Future Directions," *Advances in Wound Care* 7, no. 2 (February 1, 2018): 29–45, https://doi.org/10.1089/wound.2016.0696.

2. A. Bayat, D. A. McGrouther, and M. W. J. Ferguson, "Skin Scarring," *British Medical Journal* 326, no. 7380 (January 11, 2003): 88–92, https://doi.org/10.1136/bmj.326.7380.88.

3. Dani Di Placido, "Should Villains with Facial Scars Disappear from the Screen?" *Forbes*, November 30, 2018, https://www.forbes.com/sites /danidiplacido/2018/11/30/should-villains-with-facial-scars-disappear -from-the-screen/#6ac49fa77122.

4. J. K. Rowling, *Harry Potter and the Sorcerer's Stone* (New York: Scholastic, 1998).

5. Julian of Norwich, *Revelation of Love* (New York: Doubleday, 1997), 55.

6. Quoted in Louis Cozolino, *Attachment-Based Teaching: Creating a Tribal Classroom* (New York: W. W. Norton, 2014), 105.

7. Yousra Attia, "Photo Series Celebrates the Beauty and the Story Behind the Scars," *Elle*, October 19, 2018, https://www.elle.com/culture/a23869599 /photo-series-celebrates-the-beauty-and-the-story-behind-the-scars/.

CHAPTER 8: IN THE BEGINNING

1. This research led Bem's laboratory team to publish the following study: J. Desai et al., "*Nell1*-Deficient Mice Have Reduced Expression of Extracellular Matrix Proteins Causing Cranial and Vertebral Defects," *Human Molecular Genetics* 15, no. 8 (April 15, 2006): 1329–41, https:// doi.org/10.1093/hmg/ddl053.

2. Kerry Jamieson, "Epigenetics and ACEs," Center for Child Counseling, April 23, 2019, https://www.centerforchildcounseling.org/epigenetics -and-aces/.

3. Brené Brown, *Daring Greatly: How the Courage to Be Vulnerable Transforms the Way We Live, Love, Parent, and Lead* (New York: Avery Publishing Group, 2015), chapter 2.

4. Brown, *Daring Greatly*.

5. "Women Encircle a Crying Mom Whose Toddler Was Having a Meltdown at the Airport," Good News Network, February 15, 2018, https://www .goodnewsnetwork.org/women-encircle-crying-mom-whose-toddler -meltdown-airport/.

6. Nicole Sheinzok, "Mom Becomes Internet Villain after Toddler Terrorizes 8-Hour Flight," *Working Mother*, February 15, 2018, https://www.working mother.com/mom-becomes-internet-villain-after-toddler-terrorizes-8-hour -flight.

7. Andrew Schneider, "Biden to Meet with George Floyd's Family ahead of Houston Funeral," Houston Public Media, June 8, 2020, https://www .houstonpublicmedia.org/articles/news/2020/06/08/375357/biden-comes -to-houston-to-meet-with-floyds-family-ahead-of-funeral/.

8. See Galatians 3:28.

9. "Howard Thurman" from *This Far by Faith*, PBS, http://www.pbs.org/thisfarbyfaith/people/howard_thurman.html.
10. Howard Thurman, *Footprints of a Dream: The Story of the Church for the Fellowship of All Peoples* (Eugene, OR: Wipf and Stock, 2009), 7.
11. Jeannie Roberts, "Mother Reaches Out, Forgives Son's Killer," *Arkansas Democrat Gazette*, January 24, 2016, https://www.arkansasonline.com/news/2016/jan/24/mother-reaches-out-forgives-son-s-kille/.

CHAPTER 9: MIND AND BODY AS ONE
1. J. Dennis Mull and Dorothy S. Mull, "A Visit with a Curandero," *Western Journal of Medicine* 139, no. 5 (November 1983): 730–36, https://pubmed.ncbi.nlm.nih.gov/6659503/.
2. Mull and Mull, "A Visit with a Curandero."
3. Huseyin Guducuoglu, Serap Gunes Bilgili, and Mehmet Arslan, "Believing (Faith or Hypnosis) That Impacts on the Healing of Warts Performed by Neurophysiological Mediators," *Medical Science and Discovery* 2, no. 4 (August 2015): 236–38, https://doi.org/10.17546/msd.59888; Evren M. Hoşrik, Aydın E. Cüceloğlu, and Seval Erpolat. "Therapeutic Effects of Islamic Intercessory Prayer on Warts," *Journal of Religion and Health* 56 (December 2017): 2053–60, https://doi.org/10.1007/s10943-014-9837-z.
4. Jo Marchant, *Cure: A Journey into the Science of Mind Over Body* (New York: Crown, 2017).
5. Marchant, *Cure.*
6. S. Guo and L. A. Dipietro, "Factors Affecting Wound Healing," *Journal of Dental Research* 89, no. 3 (March 2010): 219–29, https://doi.org/10.1177/0022034509359125.
7. Courtney E. Detillion et al., "Social Facilitation of Wound Healing," *Psychoneuroendocrinology* 29, no. 8 (September 2004): 1004–11, https://doi.org/10.1016/j.psyneuen.2003.10.003.
8. K. A. Wientjes, "Mind-Body Techniques in Wound Healing." *Ostomy/Wound Management* 48, no. 11 (November 2002): 62–67, PMID: 12426453.
9. Laura Porter, Kimberly Martin, and Robert Anda, "Self-Healing Communities: A Transformational Process Model for Improving Intergenerational Health," report from the Robert Wood Johnson Foundation, June 29, 2016, https://criresilient.org/wp-content/uploads/2018/07/Self-healing-community-report.pdf.
10. Porter, Martin, and Anda, "Self-Healing Communities," 4.
11. "Our Founder, Father Greg," Homeboy Industries website, accessed December 21, 2020, https://homeboyindustries.org/our-story/father-greg/.

12. "An Evening with Greg Boyle: Healing Communities through Kinship," *America*, April 2, 2019, https://www.youtube.com/watch?v=A6xA4vdo8hw &t=4268s. See also "Homeboy," Homeboy Industries, 2019, https:// homeboyindustries.org.

13. "An Evening with Greg Boyle."

14. See John 13:23.

15. See Mark 3:17.

16. See John 3:16, the epistle 1 John; and Revelation chapters 3, 4, 5, and 21.

17. See Galatians 5:22-23.

18. J. P. Moreland, *Finding Quiet: My Story of Overcoming Anxiety and the Practices That Brought Peace* (Grand Rapids, MI: Zondervan, 2019).

CHAPTER 10: HISTORIES AND POTENTIALS

1. See Luke 5:17-26.

2. See Luke 22:19-20; John 19:28-37.

3. Hector Avalos, *Health Care and the Rise of Christianity* (Grand Rapids, MI: Baker Academic, 2010).

4. Timothy S. Miller, "Basil's House of Healing," *Christian History* 101 (2011), https://christianhistoryinstitute.org/magazine/article/basils -house-of-healing.

5. Richard Rohr, "Initiation," Center for Action and Contemplation, August 9, 2018, https://cac.org/initiation-2018-08-09.

6. Colossians 1:24, MSG.

ABOUT THE AUTHORS

Jennie Anderson McLaurin is a public health pediatrician with degrees in medicine, public health, and theology. Her work centers on special-needs children and marginalized communities in the US and abroad, with practice sites including migrant farmworker communities, indigenous Hawaiian clinics, inner-city programs, and medical centers in India and the Dominican Republic. As a national expert in community health programs, she has traveled to every state and several territories in the US. She writes, speaks, and teaches on topics of public health, bioethics, health disparities, faithful medicine, intersections of science and faith, and issues of childhood.

Additionally, she writes and teaches for faith communities—her award-winning creative nonfiction essays on the spiritual life have been published in several North American periodicals. As the recipient of a prestigious John Templeton Foundation grant, she and Cymbeline Culiat have led pastors across North America to examine the ways in which science is a friend to faith. Jennie spent three years at Regent College (Vancouver, British Columbia), serving as dean of students and as a faculty member in bioethics.

An avid hiker, Jennie is intrigued by the imprints of the Trinity found in all that we see in nature and humanity. She is drawn to further exploring how God is revealed in the world, and how those signposts can help us flourish in all the places we find ourselves. Jennie and her husband, Andrew, live in northwest Washington State with an assortment of their five young adult children.

Cymbeline (Bem) Tancongco Culiat is a scientist, entrepreneur, and educator. She is an expert in the genetic and molecular basis of mammalian development, diseases, and disorders. From 1999 to 2009, she was a senior scientist at Oak Ridge National Laboratory in Tennessee, a leading federal research institution. She discovered the role of the NELL1 signaling protein in tissue growth and maturation of the musculoskeletal and cardiovascular systems. Bem is the inventor on twenty-three patents in eight countries on the applications of the NELL1 protein in tissue regeneration. In 2020, she used improvements in the technology to co-invent its application as a therapy to heal the severe lung and heart tissue damage incurred by patients during viral infections like COVID-19. She is currently working with an international team to develop and take this treatment from the laboratory to the clinic.

In 2008, Bem cofounded NellOne Therapeutics Inc.,

a biotechnology company dedicated to pioneering products for tissue regeneration after severe injuries. In 2018, Bem cofounded Liora LLC (formerly ZoeVet), which is harnessing the NELL1 technology for veterinary products.

Bem is also a creative and dedicated teacher. For ten years she taught genetics as well as cell and molecular biology at the University of the Philippines, where she earned a bachelor's degree in cell biology and a master's degree in genetics. Bem received a PhD in biomedical sciences from the Oak Ridge National Laboratory–University of Tennessee. She completed postdoctoral training in molecular genetics and genomics there during the Human Genome Project and served as an adjunct professor of genome sciences and technology at the University of Tennessee (Knoxville) for ten years. She also mentored young scientists from high school, college, and graduate levels in her laboratory. Bem continues to lecture as an invited speaker at selected private and public universities. She is widely recognized for her work with major awards in the fields of molecular biology and genetics.

Bem has a passion for bringing the world of science to people of faith so that they can encounter wonder and wisdom in its contributions to our human understanding. She lives with her husband, Julio, and their son, Caleb, in Oak Ridge, Tennessee, where she is active in the community and church.

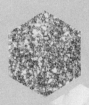